THE EARS, NOSE & THROAT

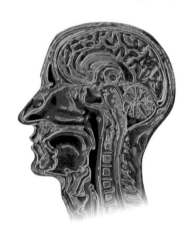

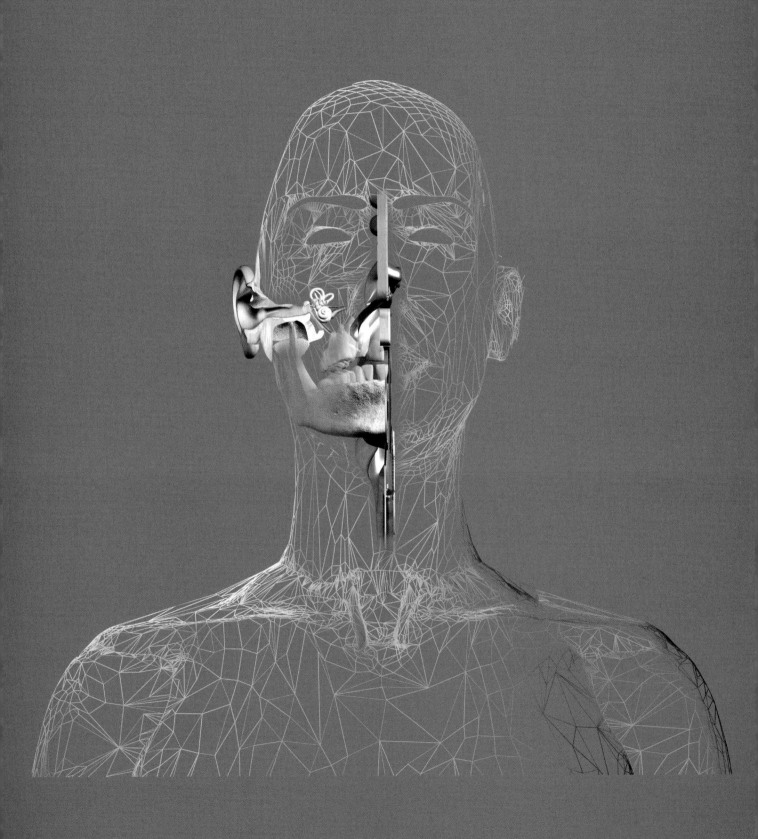

YOUR BODY YOUR HEALTH

THE
EARS, NOSE
&THROAT

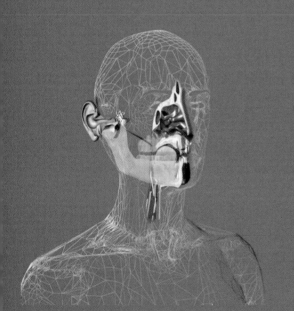
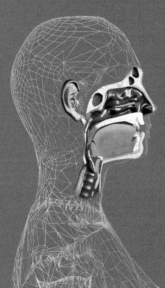
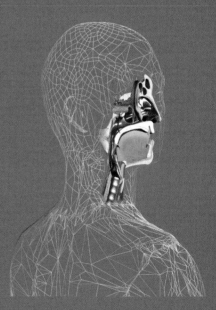

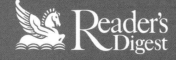
Reader's Digest

The Reader's Digest Association Limited
London New York Sydney Montreal

The Ears, Nose and Throat

was created and produced by
Carroll & Brown Limited
20 Lonsdale Road
London NW6 6RD
for Reader's Digest, London

ISBN 0 276 42700 9

Reproduced by Colourscan, Singapore
Printed and bound by Printer Industria
Gráfica S. A., Barcelona

The information in this book is for reference only; it is not intended as a substitute for a doctor's diagnosis and care. The editors urge anyone with continuing medical problems or symptoms to consult a doctor.

Managing editor
Anne Yelland

Managing art editor
Anne Fisher, Tracy Timson

Editors
Judy Fovargue, Susan McLeish, Anna Southgate

Art editors
Maxine Lea, Vimit Punater

Design assistant
Justin Ford

Series medical consultant
Dr Lesley Hickin, MB BS, BSc, DRCOG, MRCGP, General Practitioner

ENT specialist consultant
Mr Charles East, FRCS, Consultant Otolaryngologist – Head and Neck Surgeon,
Royal National Throat, Nose and Ear Hospital, Royal Free Hampstead NHS Trust, London

CONTRIBUTORS

Wynnie Chan, BSc, PhD, Public Health Nutritionist

Mr Paul Chatrath, MA (Cantab), MB BS, MRCS, DLO, Specialist Registrar in
Otolaryngology, Royal National Throat, Nose and Ear Hospital, London

Suzy Chiazzari, MIAC, MEDA, MIAHD, MASC, Interior Designer, Stress Consultant and
Colour Therapist

Jayne Comins, MSc, MRCSLT, PG Cert (Voice), Consultant Speech and Language Therapist

Miss Laura Harding, MB BS, FRCS (ORL-HNS), Specialist Registrar in Otolaryngology,
Royal National Throat, Nose and Ear Hospital, London

Dr Lesley Hickin, MB BS, BSc, DRCOG, MRCGP, General Practitioner

Mr Ben Hartley, MB BS, FRCS (ORL-HNS), Consultant Paediatric ENT Surgeon,
Great Ormond Street Hospital for Children, London

Joel Levy, BSc, MA, Medical Writer

Mr S K Lloyd, BSc (Hons), MRCS, Department of Otolaryngology,
Charing Cross Hospital, London

Amanda Sandford, Research Manager, Action on Smoking and Health

Mr David Whinney, FRCS (ORL-HNS), Consultant Ear Nose and Throat Surgeon,
The Royal Cornwall Hospital, Truro

For Reader's Digest
Series Editor Christine Noble
Art Editor Julie Bennett
Editorial Assistant Lucy Murray
Reader's Digest General Books
Editorial Director Cortina Butler
Art Director Nick Clark

The Ears, Nose and Throat

Awareness of health issues and expectations of medicine are greater today than ever before. A long and healthy life has come to be looked on as not so much a matter of luck but as almost a right. However, as our knowledge of health and the causes of disease has grown, it has become increasingly clear that health is something that we can all influence, for better or worse, through choices we make in our lives. *Your Body Your Health* is designed to help you make the right choices to make the most of your health potential. Each volume in the series focuses on a different physiological system of the body, explaining what it does and how it works. There is a wealth of advice and health tips on diet, exercise and lifestyle factors, as well as the health checks you can expect throughout life. You will find out what can go wrong and what can be done about it, and learn from people's real-life experiences of diagnosis and treatment. Finally, there is a detailed A to Z index of the major conditions which can affect the system. The series builds into a complete user's manual for the care and maintenance of the entire body.

This volume looks at the inter-related structures and functions of the ears, nose and throat. Follow a sound from the outside world to the auditory centre of your brain, and find out why the smell of freshly roasted coffee can evoke memories. Grasp the mechanics of the balance system – and why a rollercoaster ride can leave you literally not knowing which way is up. Find out how to keep your ears, nose and throat working well, and discover how simple self-help measures can help you to cope with common infections affecting the ears, nose and throat. You may be surprised at how easy it is to put your voice under stress and how social habits can adversely affect these delicate organs. Read about what you can do to safeguard ENT health against atmospheric threats like noise, and domestic threats such as dust mites. And find out about the ENT specialists, the tests that help them to identify problems, and the treatment options available, from drugs to surgery and hearing aids to speech therapy.

Contents

3

What happens when things go wrong

The ENT life story

Your ears, nose and throat are responsible for much of your communication and interaction with the world around you. The senses of hearing and smell are essential not only to your enjoyment of life and appreciation of the world, but also to your very survival, while your throat produces the sounds that enable you to make your thoughts and feelings clear to others.

At first glance the common link between the ears, nose and throat is far from obvious, and their primary functions – hearing and balance, smelling and speaking – may seem widely disparate. But despite the evident differences in their overall structures and functions, these organs and tissues are intimately linked in several ways.

The ears, nose and throat are anatomically connected by a narrow passage, known as the pharyngotympanic tube, as a result of which a disease that affects one will often affect the others, so that a single branch of medicine – known as otorhinolaryngology – covers the treatment of all three. They have a developmental connection, since all three derive from similar parts of the fetus, and they share a common degree of sensitivity – the ability to produce or detect incredibly small variations within an extremely wide range of possibilities.

These subtle distinctions are possible because of the delicate and ingenious structures that lie at the heart of each element of the otorhinolaryngeal system.

ENT PRECISION

In the throat, the taut ligaments that make up your vocal cords act like the reed of a musical instrument, giving you the power and precision to produce a range of sounds from a whisper to a song, from a single, pure note to the complex articulations that make up language. In the ears, bones and membranes transmit sound waves to pressure-sensitive hairs that translate them into electrical signals with unparalleled sensitivity. Other structures in the ears act like gyroscopes to enable us to sense gravity and motion, and keep our balance. In the nose, millions of receptor cells are alert to odour molecules, producing a device more sensitive than the finest artificial detectors.

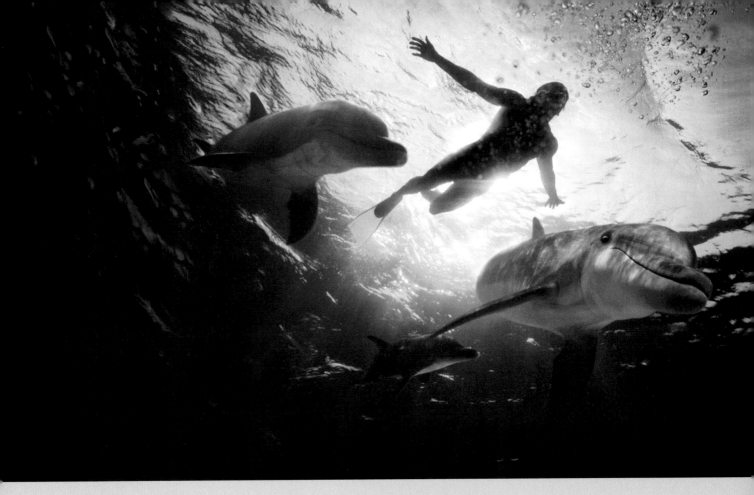

THE AQUATIC APE

The complexity and sheer ingenuity of these biological devices is a testament to the power of evolution, although the ancestral roots of some parts of the ears, nose and throat are surprising. The tiny bones of the middle ears, for instance, evolved from the gill bones of the ancient fish species that mammals evolved from, while according to one controversial theory of human evolution the specialised human larynx – the lower part of the throat that contains the vocal cords – may have originated as an adaptation to an aquatic lifestyle, rather than developing in order to facilitate speech.

The 'aquatic ape' theory argues that many aspects of human biology indicate that our earliest ancestors (the 'missing link' between us and the other types of ape) lived by the sea or large lakes and spent a lot of time immersed in water. According to this theory of evolution, the properties of the human larynx that make speech possible – its length and position in the throat, together with the ability to control breathing voluntarily – first arose in order to help early man take big gulps of air needed for diving. In other words, humans evolved diving apparatus

A common heritage?
Dolphins and other diving mammals share humans' ability to control breathing voluntarily as they dive. Although they possess no vocal cords, scientists suggest that certain species of dolphin do produce some sounds in the larynx, although most are made in the nasal sac.

first, and later generations found the adaptations useful to communicate with each other. Evidence from the ear canals of fossil Neanderthal skulls backs up this theory – they sometimes contain bony growths similar to those found in the ears of human divers.

The 'aquatic ape' theory is contentious at best. Most evolutionary biologists believe that our ability to articulate words evolved hand in hand with our ability to understand language, the one feeding off the other over tens of thousands of years. Child psychologists believe that a similar process is repeated on a much shorter timescale – about four years – every time a child learns to speak.

An especially sensitive nose can distinguish as many as 10,000 separate smells; the average person can detect perhaps half that number.

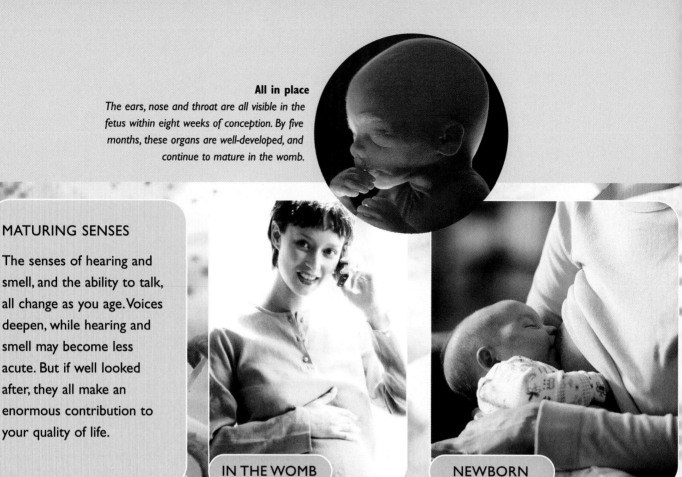

All in place
The ears, nose and throat are all visible in the fetus within eight weeks of conception. By five months, these organs are well-developed, and continue to mature in the womb.

MATURING SENSES

The senses of hearing and smell, and the ability to talk, all change as you age. Voices deepen, while hearing and smell may become less acute. But if well looked after, they all make an enormous contribution to your quality of life.

IN THE WOMB

NEWBORN

Musical memory
Recent research suggests that babies are not only able to hear music in the womb, but that 12 months later they show a clear preference for what they heard.

First things first
A baby's throat is designed for simultaneous breathing and breastfeeding, but this means they lack the ability to articulate words in the first months of life.

ENT DEVELOPMENT BEFORE BIRTH

Just days after conception, the fertilised human egg has grown into an embryo with a head-tail organisation. Within four weeks, six gill-like folds, called 'branchial arches', develop at the head end of the embryo. Each arch will become a different set of tissues in the baby – the first two become parts of the ears. Above the arches, at the 'top' of the embryo, is a mass of tissue called the fronto-nasal prominence that includes two patches of cells on its surface. These patches will develop into the olfactory lining, where the sense of smell is located. On the outside of the fronto-nasal prominence is a band of tissue that, over the next four weeks, curls up and around to form the external nose. By this time depressions have already formed inside it to give nostrils.

Meanwhile, below the branchial arches, the beginnings of the digestive system are already present in rudimentary form in the shape of a simple tube. The top of this tube will become the pharynx and a number of pouches develop from it. The first two pouches link up with the first two branchial arches to give rise to the structures of the ears, including the pharyngotympanic tube which connects the ears and throat. Meanwhile, a shallow groove in the floor of the primitive pharynx grows into the larynx. Around day 24–26 of development the nostrils join to the pharynx. By week eight the fetus has a recognisable face with ears and a nose.

Over the next seven months these structures develop, fill in and expand. Some even start functioning. A baby in the womb can hear, for instance, enabling it to recognise

Hearing and listening
Children learn language rapidly and by the age of five are using it to hold conversations, ask questions, and take turns and listen.

Sound check
As teenagers mature, the voice deepens and becomes more powerful in both boys and girls, with a full range of sounds.

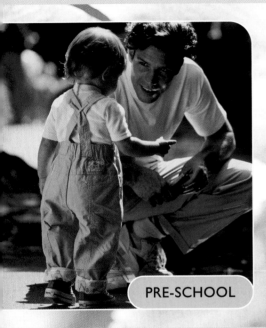

PRE-SCHOOL

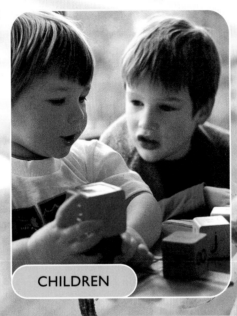

CHILDREN

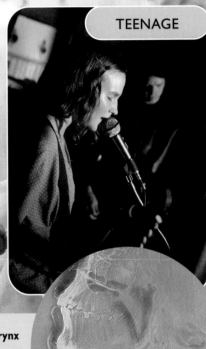

TEENAGE

Chatter chatter
Toddlers learn words at a phenomenal rate, but their still immature vocal system means that their own attempts at speaking are not wholly intelligible to others.

Lengthening larynx
At puberty, the larynx becomes longer in boys, resulting in a much deeper voice.

its mother's voice at birth. Experts believe that babies may even be able to smell in the uterus, picking up telltale maternal scent molecules in the amniotic fluid, priming them to respond to their mother's odour at birth.

At birth, a newborn baby's vocal apparatus is ready for use, enabling it to scream lustily from its first breath. A newborn, however, lacks the ability to speak even if it knew how, because its larynx is in the wrong position. For the first six months the larynx is positioned to allow a baby to breathe at the same time as breastfeeding.

FROM GURGLES TO RATTLES

In the first six months, babies are learning how to integrate the functions of their hearing and speaking apparatus. At first, they practise making noises – cooing, gurgling and laughing for three months, babbling during the following three – while at the same time learning to understand language. By six months babies have a unique ability to distinguish between word sounds they've never heard before, and although they may not speak their first words for another six months they are already acquiring, with amazing speed, the rules of grammar and syntax that underlie their mother tongue. By the age of three the average child will be learning 10 new words a day.

During childhood and puberty the structures of the ears, nose and throat change and grow. As the skull thickens the auditory canal connecting the middle ear to the outside world elongates and acquires a slight bend. The pharyngotympanic tube doubles in length, making it harder

Smell the taste
The senses of taste and smell are intrinsically linked, a fact that becomes obvious when we eat: having a blocked nose can render food tasteless.

Fragrant flowers
Although the sense of smell becomes less acute in later life, most people retain the ability to discern and enjoy an enormous number of fragrances.

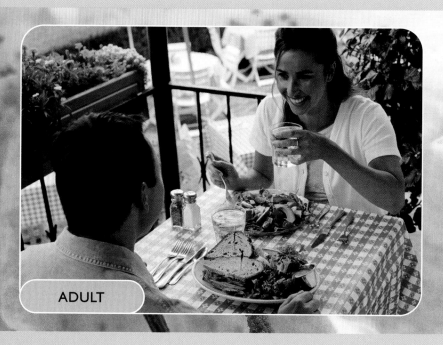

ADULT

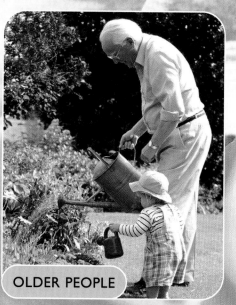

OLDER PEOPLE

for bacteria to get from the throat to the ear, so that ear infections become less common. Puberty brings a surge of hormones that affect the vocal cords. The larynx grows and the cords get longer, thicker and heavier, particularly in males. The average frequency of a child's voice is 265Hz; for an adult woman it is 225Hz and for a man a low 120Hz.

While some parts of the ear are growing, however, some are already experiencing the effects of ageing. You begin to lose sensory hairs in your inner ear from the moment you are born, causing a very gradual but real decrease in the sensitivity of your hearing. It takes longer for your nose to be affected, but eventually the olfactory sensory cells of the nose begin to thin out, making it harder for older people to detect faint odours and dulling their sense of taste. Even the vocal cords may be affected, stiffening and thinning with extreme old age, so that the voice may become reedy. The moment of death itself may be marked by a final spasm of the vocal cords, which produces the 'death rattle'.

LIFESTYLE AND ENT HEALTH
Day-to-day health issues can also affect the functioning of the vocal cords. A cold can cause swelling and inflammation, leading to hoarseness or even temporary paralysis of the cords. Lifestyle choices such as smoking have a major influence on the incidence and severity of such infections, and on the health of other parts of your ears, nose and throat. Making positive lifestyle choices, including not smoking, avoiding noise and air pollution as far as possible, taking exercise, learning to deal with stress and adopting a healthy diet can have profound short and long-term effects on your otorhinolaryngeal health.

In the long term, a healthy lifestyle can help to improve and preserve the sensitivity of your palate and your enjoyment of the subtleties of music and speech, and can be a major contributor to your quality of life. The protective effects of a healthy lifestyle are also important in the short term, as problems affecting your ears, nose and throat, while not necessarily life-threatening, are

The composer Beethoven suffered from the degenerative disease otosclerosis, which today can be treated by surgery or alleviated with a hearing aid.

among the most irritating and frequently encountered. Ear infections, for instance, are extremely common childhood ailments, which, if poorly managed, can have long-term implications for hearing. Hay fever and other forms of allergy are becoming increasingly common, and colds and flu infections are not simply regular nuisances – they pose a real risk to the elderly and vulnerable.

Awareness, a healthy lifestyle and simple preventative measures can help you to avoid or minimise many ear, nose and throat problems, while modern medicine has developed a battery of treatments, from the traditional, such as removal of the tonsils, to the advanced, such as cochlear implants ('bionic' inner ear components). Some aspects of ear, nose and throat medicine have become routine – drug therapies for hay fever, for instance, are now widely available as over-the-counter medicines.

ENT AND THE FUTURE

In the present day a lot of otorhinolaryngeal medicine focuses on management of problems rather than cure or prevention, but in the future we may see exciting new avenues of treatment. Short-term prospects include improved flu and cold vaccinations, treatments for motion sickness and radically improved hearing aids.

Further into the future such technology might be applied to the healthy ear, enhancing normal hearing by selecting what to amplify and what to filter out, helping to combat noise pollution. 'Smart' hearing aids might even be able to translate normally inaudible sounds, or other forms of environmental information, into audible sounds. One day you might be able to 'hear' your partner's heart beat or your child's temperature. Similar technology, applied in reverse, might be used to enhance and alter voices, so that everyone could become an accomplished singer, or to modify the sense of smell so that you could pick up scents that are normally undetectable.

Such bionic senses are a long way off, and many would argue that they are unnecessary for healthy men and women. The human voice is already capable of a fantastic range of expression, and the amazing structures of your ears and nose have the potential to provide a constantly rich and dazzling sensory feast – as long as you look after them.

The future of sound
These jagged white waveforms represent voice patterns produced by a voice-recognition computer. Developments in speech synthesis may help those who have to have their voice box removed.

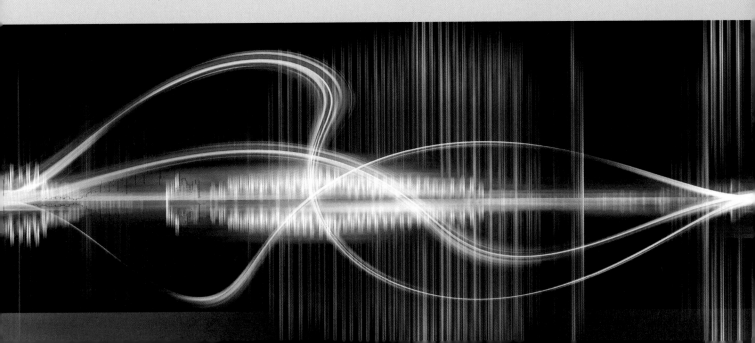

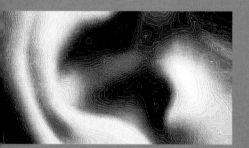
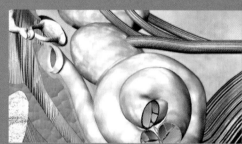
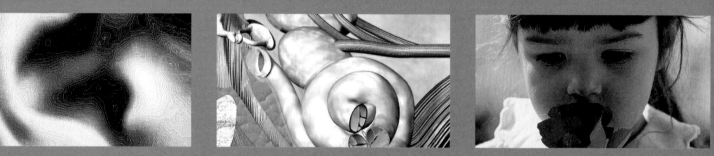

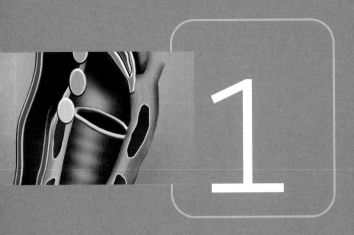

1

How your ears, nose and throat work

Your amazing ears, nose and throat

Talking, hearing, smelling, standing upright – these are abilities we usually take for granted. But the structures they depend on are some of the greatest marvels in the human body.

The inner ear *contains the structures needed for hearing and balance. For more information on how they work, see pages 24–25 and pages 26–27.*

The middle ear *contains tiny bones that are so sensitive they can transmit the sound of a pin dropping. Find out how they cope with both loud and quiet noises on pages 20–21.*

THE MULTIFUNCTIONAL EARS, NOSE AND THROAT

Your ears, nose and throat are an interconnected system of chambers, passages and extraordinarily complex sensory organs. Between them these structures perform several major functions – swallowing, the production of sound, the sensation of balance, hearing and smell – and a host of minor ones. Smelling, technically known as olfaction, is done by part of the lining of your nasal cavity (the space inside your nose) and your brain. This space opens out into your pharynx and larynx, which together make up your throat, where speech and other sound is produced. A narrow tube – the eustachian tube – connects the air spaces of your nose and throat to the air spaces of your ear, where the structures of hearing and balance sensation are located. The ear itself has three regions: the outer, middle and inner ear.

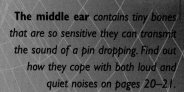

Purposeful pinna
The outer, visible part of your ear is called the pinna. It may not look very useful, but it plays an important role in your hearing; see pages 18–19.

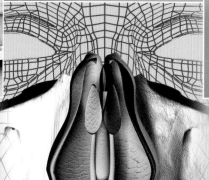

What's in a nose?
The external structure of your nose is made up of skin, bone and cartilage. Find out how they fit together on pages 28–29.

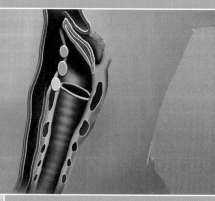

In the pipeline
The throat is more than a delivery hatch for food, drink and air – it also produces sound, enabling you to speak and sing. Turn to pages 34–35 to find out how.

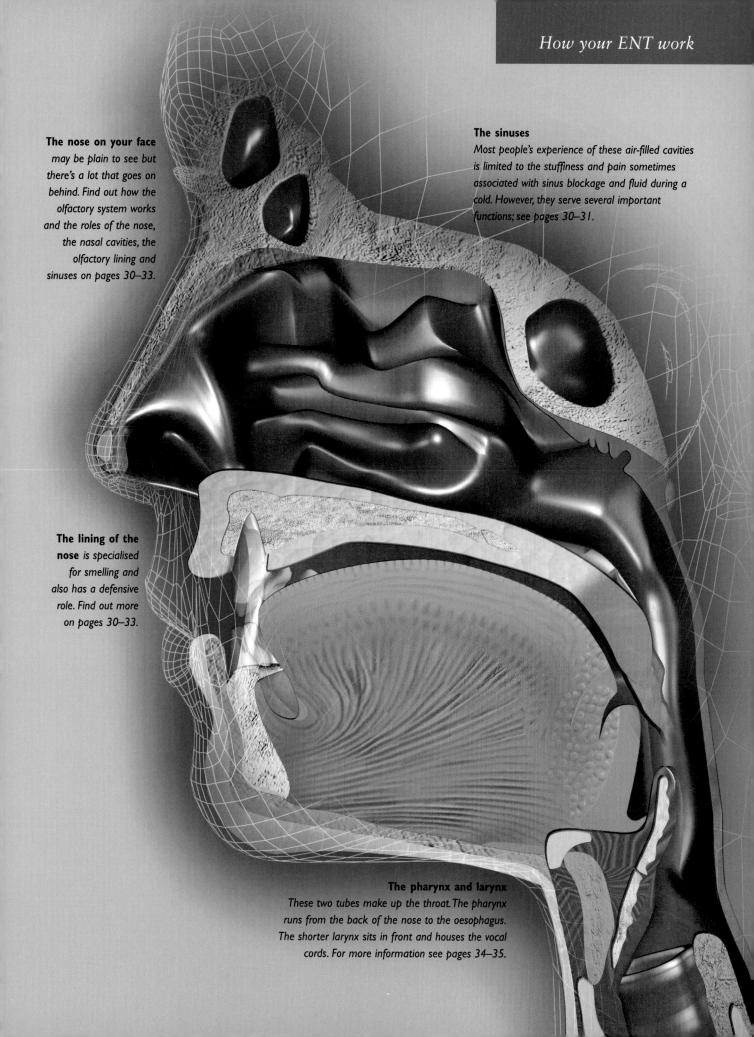

The nose on your face *may be plain to see but there's a lot that goes on behind. Find out how the olfactory system works and the roles of the nose, the nasal cavities, the olfactory lining and sinuses on pages 30–33.*

The sinuses
Most people's experience of these air-filled cavities is limited to the stuffiness and pain sometimes associated with sinus blockage and fluid during a cold. However, they serve several important functions; see pages 30–31.

The lining of the nose *is specialised for smelling and also has a defensive role. Find out more on pages 30–33.*

The pharynx and larynx
These two tubes make up the throat. The pharynx runs from the back of the nose to the oesophagus. The shorter larynx sits in front and houses the vocal cords. For more information see pages 34–35.

The outer ear

The outer portion of the ear has several important functions, without which your hearing would be compromised. It collects sound and directs it to the inner ear, and it helps to protect the delicate structures inside the ear from the outside world.

In men, outer ear tissue continues to grow, so older men have larger pinnae than younger men.

EAR APPARENT

Most of your complex hearing apparatus is hidden away inside your skull, its fragile components shielded by a wall of solid bone. These inner portions are connected to the outside world by a short passage called the auditory canal. The inner end of the canal terminates in a sheet of membrane called the eardrum, while the entrance to the canal is guarded by the visible, outer part of the ear – the pinna.

The sound collector

The pinna, also known as the auricle, is a flap of cartilage and flesh. Apart from providing a physical barrier to foreign objects that might get into the ear, its primary function is to collect sound, like a satellite dish collects television signals, and direct it to the auditory canal.

The helix is the outer, curved, fleshy ridge of the pinna.

Auditory canal

The concha is the cavity around which the antihelix curves.

The antihelix is the curved inner ridge of the pinna.

The mastoid process is a knob of bone that is the point of attachment for various muscles of the neck.

Cartilage runs through the pinna, giving it flexibility and strength.

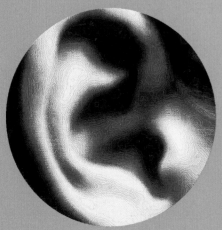

Ear exterior
The folds and grooves of the pinna are not there just by chance – they modify the transmission of sound waves to the middle and inner ear in a way that helps the brain to determine the location of the sound source.

The ear lobe is the fleshy lower portion of the pinna.

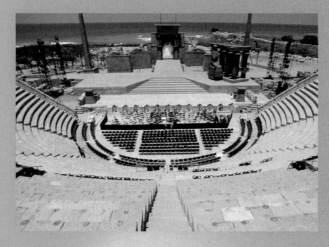

Collecting sound
In some ways, the pinna is the reverse of an amphitheatre. An amphitheatre is designed to amplify sound from the centre – the stage – and distribute it so that it can be heard even along the theatre's topmost rim, whereas the pinna collects sound from the world around it and funnels it towards the middle ear.

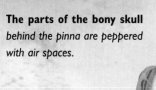

The parts of the bony skull
behind the pinna are peppered with air spaces.

Eardrum

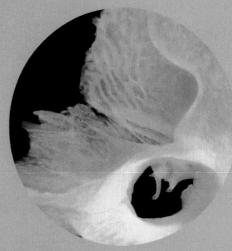

The auditory canal
The bony parts of the skull behind the pinna are shown in this coloured X-ray. The auditory canal that leads to the middle ear is visible at bottom right.

HEARING CANAL

In an adult, the auditory canal is about 2.5cm (1in) long. The walls of the outer third are made up of flesh and cartilage, while the inner two-thirds are flesh bound tightly to bone – so tightly that any swelling or inflammation in this zone causes extreme tension and therefore pain. Hairs help to prevent large particles getting into the canal, and glands in the outer part and on the pinna produce wax. There are more than 400 wax glands in each ear. Earwax traps particles before they can get too far into the canal, helps to slow down the growth of bacteria and protects the canal from becoming waterlogged when water gets into it.

Nerves of the auditory canal

The nerves that supply the auditory canal have the same root as nerves that connect to the airways, stomach and heart, which is why irritation of the canal, during syringing for instance, can lead to coughing and sneezing, and vomiting in children. The nerves of the auditory canal may be the site of pain from another part of the system, such as a tooth or the tonsils.

The middle ear

The tiny space of the middle ear houses a miniature biological sound system that can outperform any stereo for accuracy of sound reproduction, range of tones and amplifying power.

DRUM KIT

The middle ear is a space about 15mm wide, 15mm deep and 4mm high (⅗ x ⅗ x ⅙in) – about the size of a Scrabble letter. Suspended inside this cavity are three bones called the malleus, incus and stapes that are collectively known as ossicles (Latin for 'little bones'). The role of the ossicles is to transmit sound from the eardrum to the inner ear, where the organs of hearing are located.

FROM AIR TO FLUID

Most of the sound that you hear travels as waves passing through the air, but in contrast to the middle ear, the sensory structures of the inner ear sit in fluid. This means that before you can register the sound waves they have to transfer from air to fluid. Usually this sort of transfer would result in a loss of energy, making the sound waves much harder to pick up, so the middle ear works to magnify the intensity of sound as it passes from the eardrum, through the ossicles, to the oval window. It does this through a simple trick: the oval window is 22 times smaller than the ear drum, so that the displacement of the eardrum caused by an arriving sound wave is concentrated and thereby magnified 22 times when it is transmitted to the oval window.

BANGING THE DRUM

Your eardrum works like a drum in reverse. In a real drum, a taut sheet of material produces sound waves when struck with a stick. In your eardrum, sound waves from the air strike the taut sheet of membrane, making it vibrate. The vibrations pass to the handle of the malleus, which transmits them on to the incus, and then the stapes. The footplate of the stapes presses down, making the oval window to the inner ear bulge inward.

A NATURAL EQUALISER

To allow faithful transmission of sound from the eardrum to the oval window, the pressure inside the middle ear must be equal to the pressure in the auditory canal and the rest of the outside world. However, the eardrum makes an airtight seal between the two. To get round this, the middle ear connects to the back of the throat via the 36mm (1½in) long eustachian tube. When you swallow, this tube briefly opens, allowing air to pass in and out of the middle ear and automatically equalising the pressure on either side of the eardrum.

The ossicles

The three ossicles are named individually in Latin after the tools they resemble: malleus means hammer, incus is Latin for anvil and stapes (pictured below) means stirrup. They are the three tiniest bones in the body: the malleus is just 8mm (⅓in) long, and the incus and stirrup are of similar size. Our ossicles are descended, via reptilian jaw bones, from the gill bones of primordial fish.

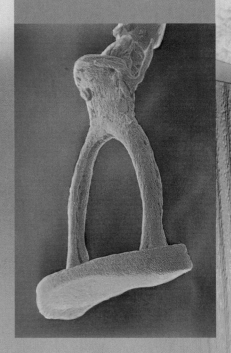

It takes less than one tenth of a second for the muscles attached to the ossicles to tense in reflex to a loud sound.

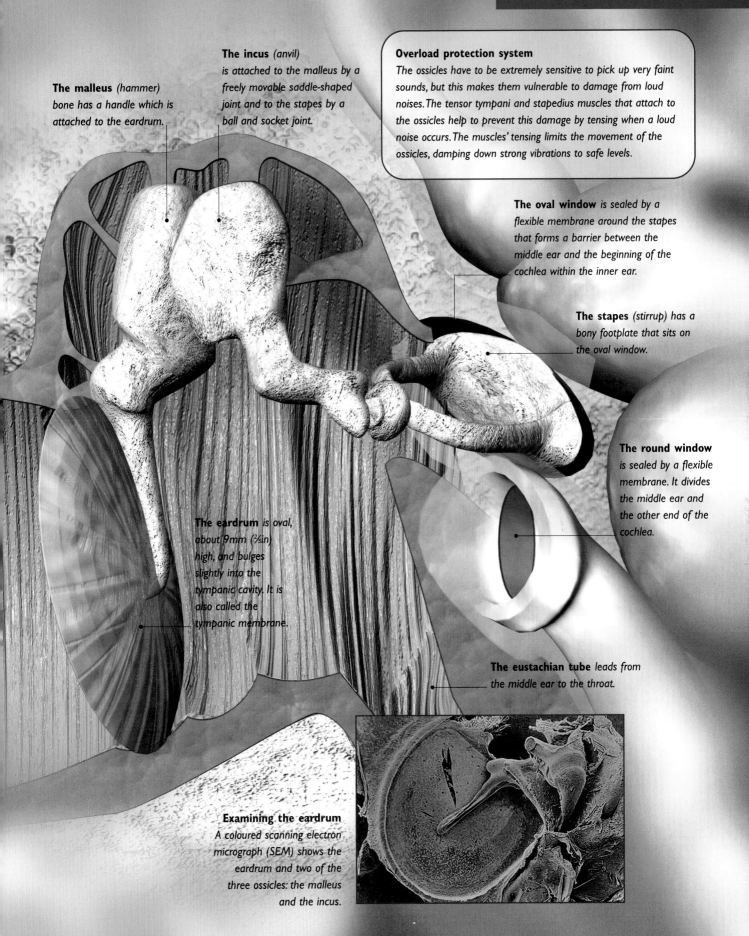

The malleus *(hammer) bone has a handle which is attached to the eardrum.*

The incus *(anvil) is attached to the malleus by a freely movable saddle-shaped joint and to the stapes by a ball and socket joint.*

Overload protection system
The ossicles have to be extremely sensitive to pick up very faint sounds, but this makes them vulnerable to damage from loud noises. The tensor tympani and stapedius muscles that attach to the ossicles help to prevent this damage by tensing when a loud noise occurs. The muscles' tensing limits the movement of the ossicles, damping down strong vibrations to safe levels.

The oval window *is sealed by a flexible membrane around the stapes that forms a barrier between the middle ear and the beginning of the cochlea within the inner ear.*

The stapes *(stirrup) has a bony footplate that sits on the oval window.*

The eardrum *is oval, about 9mm (⅜in) high, and bulges slightly into the tympanic cavity. It is also called the tympanic membrane.*

The round window *is sealed by a flexible membrane. It divides the middle ear and the other end of the cochlea.*

The eustachian tube *leads from the middle ear to the throat.*

Examining the eardrum
A coloured scanning electron micrograph (SEM) shows the eardrum and two of the three ossicles: the malleus and the incus.

The inner ear

On either side of your skull – about 4cm (1⅜in) from the outside – are the bony labyrinths, where the energy of sound waves, gravity or head movements are translated into nervous impulses for your brain to interpret.

ENTER THE LABYRINTH

The inner ear's bony labyrinth is a series of bony tubes that coil and interconnect. Inside this hard shell, following its twists and turns, is a set of fluid-filled, tube-shaped, membranous sacs called the membranous labyrinth. Inside the membranous labyrinth are the structures that translate inputs such as the direction of gravity or the frequency of a sound wave into nerve impulses. The bony labyrinth has three main components: the vestibule, the semicircular canals and the cochlea.

HAIRS OF HEARING

The three parts of the inner ear use different structures to perform their varied sensory tasks, but all rely on the same underlying mechanism – the translation of physical movement into a nerve impulse. This is performed by hair cells, which are found in all three parts of the inner ear. A hair cell is a specialised sensory cell. At its top, tiny hairs called stereocilia and kinocilia stick out. At its base, the hair cell connects to the nervous system. Movement of the hairs, such as by a passing sound wave, causes chemical changes in the cell membrane surrounding the hair. These changes in turn cause the hair cell to fire off a nerve impulse from its base.

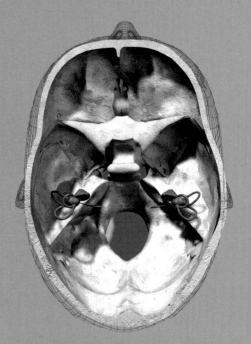

The bony labyrinths
The location of the bony labyrinths within a human skull are shown above. The outline of the outer ears can be seen on either side, with the nose at the top.

Inside the cochlea
A computed tomography (CT) scan reveals an interior cross-section through one turn of the cochlea.

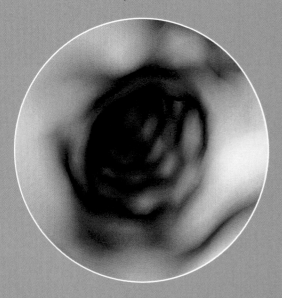

Liquid centre

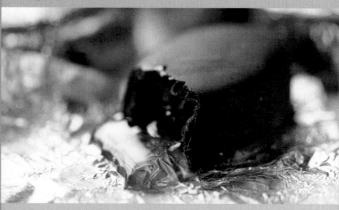

The membranous labyrinth is filled with a type of fluid called endolymph, and surrounded by a different fluid called perilymph. Endolymph has special properties that enhance the sensitivity of the hair cells. It contains high levels of electrolytes, which cause the hair cells to be more easily triggered by tiny movements.

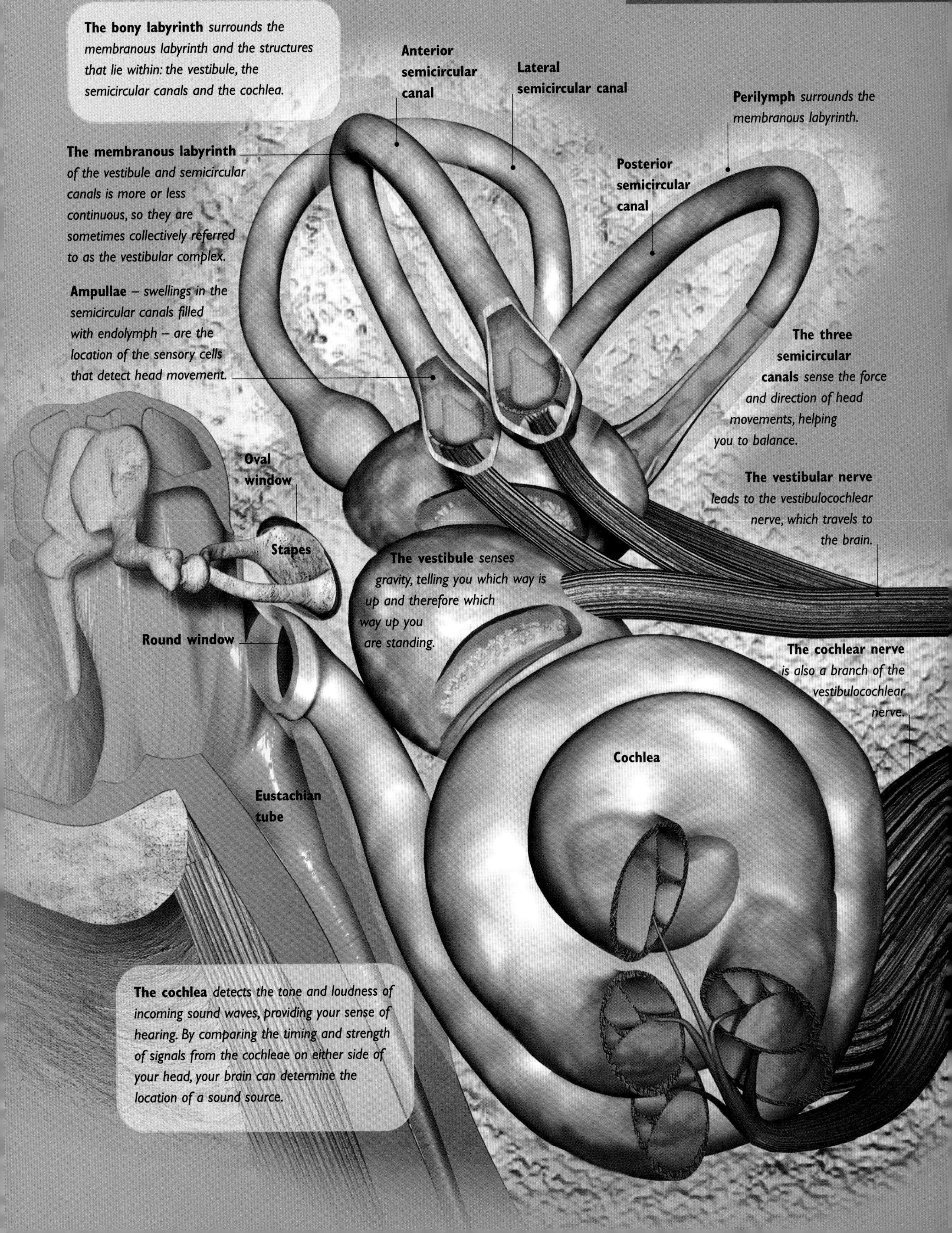

The bony labyrinth *surrounds the membranous labyrinth and the structures that lie within: the vestibule, the semicircular canals and the cochlea.*

Anterior semicircular canal

Lateral semicircular canal

Perilymph *surrounds the membranous labyrinth.*

Posterior semicircular canal

The membranous labyrinth *of the vestibule and semicircular canals is more or less continuous, so they are sometimes collectively referred to as the vestibular complex.*

Ampullae *– swellings in the semicircular canals filled with endolymph – are the location of the sensory cells that detect head movement.*

The three **semicircular canals** *sense the force and direction of head movements, helping you to balance.*

Oval window

The vestibular nerve *leads to the vestibulocochlear nerve, which travels to the brain.*

Stapes

The vestibule *senses gravity, telling you which way is up and therefore which way up you are standing.*

Round window

The cochlear nerve *is also a branch of the vestibulocochlear nerve.*

Cochlea

Eustachian tube

The cochlea *detects the tone and loudness of incoming sound waves, providing your sense of hearing. By comparing the timing and strength of signals from the cochleae on either side of your head, your brain can determine the location of a sound source.*

Hearing

The cochlea within the inner ear contains the hearing apparatus which is able to sense the two defining aspects of sound – frequency, also known as pitch, and loudness, also known as amplitude.

SOUND IN THE ROUND

The cochlea is a bony coil with two-and-a-half turns. It begins at the oval window and ends at the round window; the end of the coil farthest away from these windows is called the apex. The cross-section shows that the cochlea is made up of three ducts. The top and bottom (vestibular and tympanic) ducts are filled with perilymph; they join up at cochlea's apex, so that they actually comprise a single continuous duct that starts at the oval window and finishes at the round window. The middle duct is called the cochlear duct; this is filled with endolymph and contains the Organ of Corti, where sound-sensing takes place.

SOUND DETECTION

Loudness is determined by the amount of bending and flexing that sensory stereocilia undergo. The frequency (pitch) that you hear is determined by which part of the cochlea vibrates (or resonates) most in response to an incoming sound. Lower frequency sounds resonate most at the apex of the cochlea; higher frequencies at the cochlea's base, near the cochlear nerve. The different regions of the cochlea map directly onto the part of the brain that interprets sound, so that a signal from the apex of the cochlea is translated into the sensation of hearing a low frequency sound.

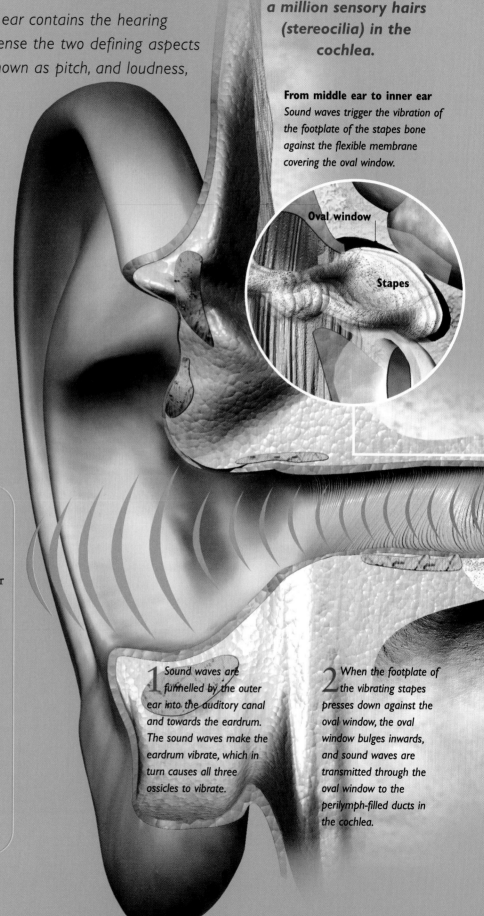

There are more than a million sensory hairs (stereocilia) in the cochlea.

From middle ear to inner ear
Sound waves trigger the vibration of the footplate of the stapes bone against the flexible membrane covering the oval window.

Oval window

Stapes

1 *Sound waves are funnelled by the outer ear into the auditory canal and towards the eardrum. The sound waves make the eardrum vibrate, which in turn causes all three ossicles to vibrate.*

2 *When the footplate of the vibrating stapes presses down against the oval window, the oval window bulges inwards, and sound waves are transmitted through the oval window to the perilymph-filled ducts in the cochlea.*

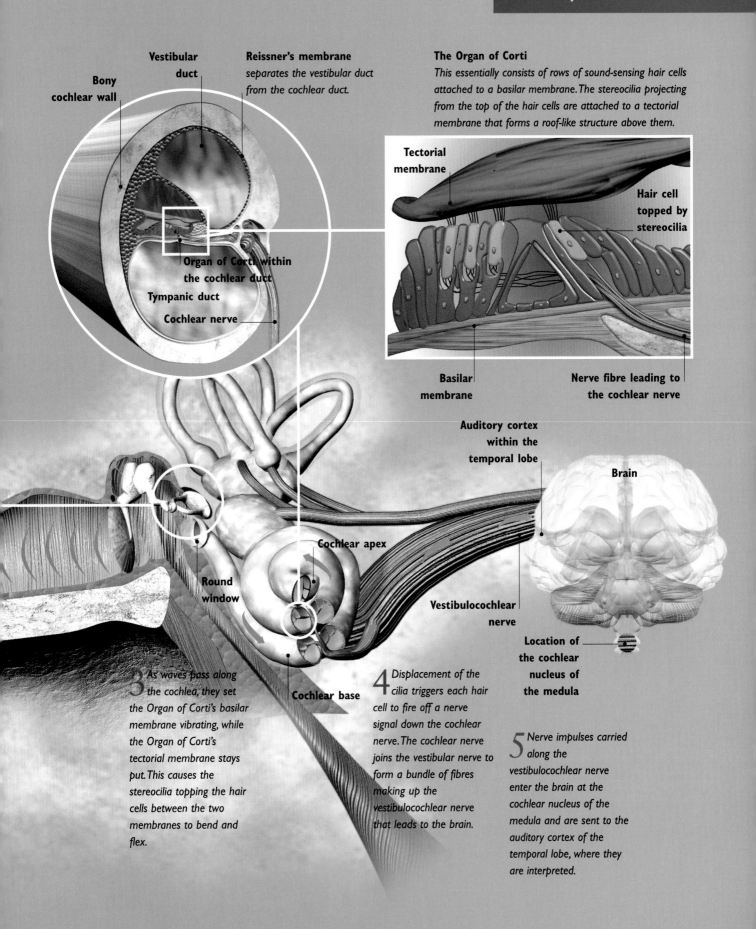

Bony cochlear wall

Vestibular duct

Reissner's membrane *separates the vestibular duct from the cochlear duct.*

The Organ of Corti
This essentially consists of rows of sound-sensing hair cells attached to a basilar membrane. The stereocilia projecting from the top of the hair cells are attached to a tectorial membrane that forms a roof-like structure above them.

Tectorial membrane

Hair cell topped by stereocilia

Organ of Corti within the cochlear duct

Tympanic duct

Cochlear nerve

Basilar membrane

Nerve fibre leading to the cochlear nerve

Auditory cortex within the temporal lobe

Brain

Cochlear apex

Round window

Vestibulocochlear nerve

Location of the cochlear nucleus of the medula

Cochlear base

3 *As waves pass along the cochlea, they set the Organ of Corti's basilar membrane vibrating, while the Organ of Corti's tectorial membrane stays put. This causes the stereocilia topping the hair cells between the two membranes to bend and flex.*

4 *Displacement of the cilia triggers each hair cell to fire off a nerve signal down the cochlear nerve. The cochlear nerve joins the vestibular nerve to form a bundle of fibres making up the vestibulocochlear nerve that leads to the brain.*

5 *Nerve impulses carried along the vestibulocochlear nerve enter the brain at the cochlear nucleus of the medula and are sent to the auditory cortex of the temporal lobe, where they are interpreted.*

Balance

Normally you only notice your sense of equilibrium when it's going wrong. But underlying this sense is a remarkable marriage of basic mechanical principles and complex, high-precision, biological engineering.

MAKING SENSE OF MOTION

In order to be able to stand up, sit down and walk around, never mind more complex manoeuvres such as a handstand, your body needs to be able to sense a number of different things: the direction of gravity, your orientation with respect to gravity, and the speed and angle of movement of your head (which controls the rest of the body). All these different components contribute to your overall sense of balance.

It is the semicircular canals (in the inner ear's bony labyrinth) that allow you to sense the motion of your head. Each ear has three canals, at right angles to each other, so you can sense movement in any plane.

DETECTING HEAD MOVEMENT

Inside the ampulla of each of your inner ear's semicircular canals is a structure called the crista. The crista is made up of hair cells on the wall of the ampulla. Tiny cilia (kinocilia and stereocilia) at the top of these hairs are embedded in a gelatinous mass called the cupula, which floats in the endolymph. When your head moves, the inertia of the cupula makes it lag slightly behind, so that it tugs on the cilia and activates the hair cells. When your head stops, the cupula overshoots slightly, tugging on the cilia in the other direction. The movement of the cilia in any direction triggers nerve impulses which are then interpreted by the brain.

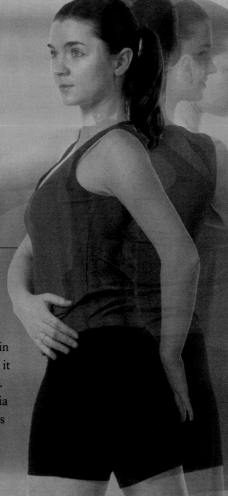

Turning sideways
When the head moves from side to side – as here – or backwards or forwards, so do hair cells in the inner ear's semicircular canals. Shifting hair cells trigger nerve impulses that keep the brain informed of the head's exact position.

A cross section of a crista *and cupula in the inner ear. The crista is the sensory structure that detects head movement.*

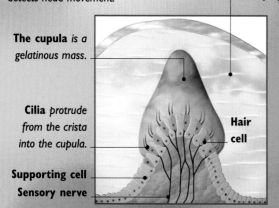

Endolymph

The cupula *is a gelatinous mass.*

Cilia *protrude from the crista into the cupula.*

Hair cell

Supporting cell
Sensory nerve

Cilia are upright when the head is still

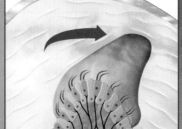

The Cupula tugs the cilia sideways as the head stops turning

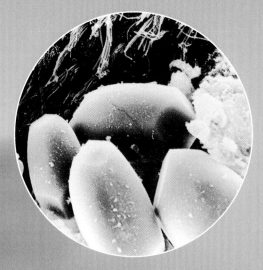

Limestone in your ears
A scanning electron microscope reveals the structure of a single otolith. Otoliths are made out of calcium carbonate, which is also found in limestone, chalk and marble.

Taking a bow
As the head bends forwards – as here – backwards or sideways, sensory hair cells of the inner ear's vestibule follow suit. This allows your brain to detect the pull of gravity when you move your head.

SENSING THE PULL OF GRAVITY

Hair cells in the vestibule component of the inner ear provide your sense of gravity. They are found in clusters called maculae within the saccule and the utricle – both parts of the membranous labyrinth inside the vestibule. As with hair cells of the semicircular canals, the cilia are embedded in a gelatinous mass, but in this case there is an added ingredient – millions of tiny mineral crystals called otoliths. Their weight provides a mass for gravity to work on. When you are standing upright, gravity presses them down, slightly squashing the cilia on the hair cells, which triggers the production of nerve impulses. If you tilt your head, the mass of otoliths slides to one side, pulling the cilia with them and sending matching nerve impulses to the brain.

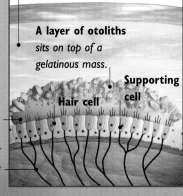

Endolymph

Cilia (stereocilia and kinocilia) *are embedded in the gelatinous mass.*

A layer of otoliths *sits on top of a gelatinous mass.*

Hair cell

Supporting cell

Sensory nerve

Cilia are upright when the head is upright

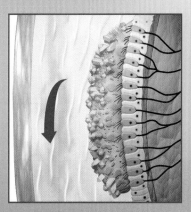

Cilia bend downwards as the head drops forward

A cross section of a macula *within the vestibule. The macula is the sensory structure that detects the pull of gravity.*

27

The nose

The visible part of your respiratory and olfactory systems is your nose. Big or small, it protects the entrance to your airways and helps you to gather samples of air for smelling.

FLESH AND BONES

The external nose is a covering of skin and flesh over a supporting framework of bone and cartilage. Pieces of cartilage provide the stiff framework that prevents the nostrils from collapsing. The inside of the nose is divided into two by the nasal septum.

NO NOSE IS BAD NOSE

The external nose serves a number of important functions.

- The cartilage and bone keep the nostrils open for easy passage of air, while nostril hairs and the ability to narrow the nostrils in response to an offensive odour (that is, wrinkle your nose) help to prevent noxious gases or foreign objects getting into the respiratory system.
- By effectively extending the respiratory and olfactory tract beyond the face, the nose allows you to sample smells from inside objects or through narrow openings – in other words, you can poke your nose into places the face cannot fit.
- Lastly, and perhaps most obviously, your nose prevents water from running into your breathing passages by shielding them from the rain, like an umbrella, or by trapping air (and thereby keeping out the water) if you need to submerge your head.

CARTILAGE AND BONE

The nasal bones *project slightly from the front of the skull. They are fused to the maxilla (the facial bone).*

Lateral cartilage *extends from the nasal bones to form the more flexible portion of your nose.*

The alar cartilages *form wings of cartilage that flank the outer edges of the nostrils.*

The accessory cartilages *lie between the lateral part of the alar cartilage and the bony nasal opening.*

Crucial underpinning
Bone and cartilage work together to provide the framework which enables the nose to perform its main function of allowing air to enter through the nostrils.

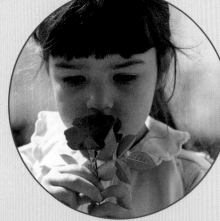

Made for smelling
Because the nose projects from the face, you can catch subtle scents that might otherwise be missed.

INSIDE THE NOSE

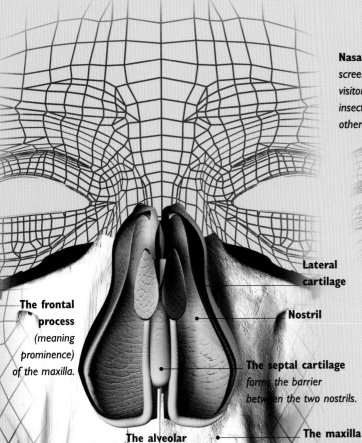

The frontal process *(meaning prominence) of the maxilla.*

Lateral cartilage

Nostril

The septal cartilage *forms the barrier between the two nostrils.*

The alveolar process *(prominence) of the maxilla.*

The maxilla – *the main facial bone – surrounds the nose on both sides and below.*

Vertical cross-section of the nose
The projecting parts of the nose have been cut away here to reveal the nostrils and septal cartilage.

Research has found that the nose may swell slightly and lengthen as a result of the stress induced by telling a lie.

LOOKING UP THE NOSTRILS

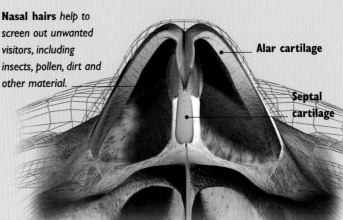

Nasal hairs *help to screen out unwanted visitors, including insects, pollen, dirt and other material.*

Alar cartilage

Septal cartilage

The lining of the two nostrils
The nostrils' lining is covered with a very delicate membrane, rich in blood vessels and nerve endings. This can be painful if it is damaged and tends to bleed easily.

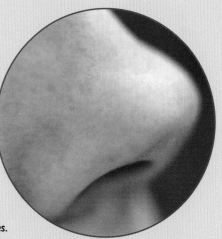

The nares – *the openings to the nostrils – are surrounded by fibro-fatty tissue, which overlays the greater alar cartilages.*

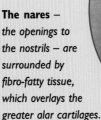

Skin protection
The vulnerable, exposed, outer skin of the nose is well supplied with tiny sebaceous glands. These secrete oil to provide a protective oily coating for the skin that keeps the skin supple and forms a barrier between the skin and the air outside.

The nasal cavity

Between the roof of your mouth and the bottom of your brain, is an irregularly shaped space known as the nasal cavity, which has important roles in respiration, smell and defending the body from illness.

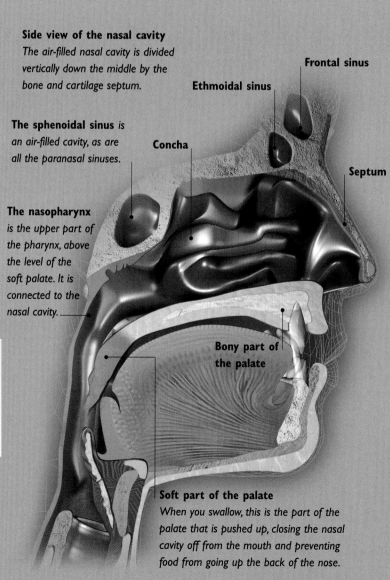

THE NASAL CAVITY

The front of the nasal cavity is connected to the outside world by the nostrils, while at the back it opens onto the top of the throat. Several smaller chambers, called sinuses, lead off from the sides. The nasal cavity's functions include olfaction (sense of smell); filtering, heating and humidifying incoming air to prevent damage to the lungs; and defence against invading micro-organisms. The cavity is mostly lined with a moist mucous membrane which produces mucus and is equipped with cilia to help carry 'dirty' mucus to the throat, where it is swallowed. In addition, the olfactory lining on the roof of the nasal cavity includes sensory receptors that respond to odour molecules, providing your sense of smell.

THE PARANASAL SINUSES

Because the various sinuses adjacent to the nasal cavity are usually filled with air, they provide resonant spaces that are important in the production of sound. Their extensive inner surfaces are lined with mucus-producing membrane, so they can generate large amounts of mucus for flushing out the nasal cavity.

The great divide
In mammals the nasal cavity and the mouth are divided by the palate, separating the digestive and olfactory systems. This allows mammals to use their sense of smell even while their mouth is full – a vital skill for prey animals such as antelope which need to be on their guard at all times.

Side view of the nasal cavity
The air-filled nasal cavity is divided vertically down the middle by the bone and cartilage septum.

The sphenoidal sinus *is an air-filled cavity, as are all the paranasal sinuses.*

Frontal sinus

Ethmoidal sinus

Concha

Septum

The nasopharynx *is the upper part of the pharynx, above the level of the soft palate. It is connected to the nasal cavity.*

Bony part of the palate

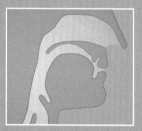

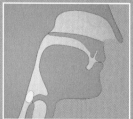

When you breathe
The soft palate is relaxed, allowing air inhaled via the mouth to move freely into the nasopharynx and the nasal cavity.

When you swallow
The soft palate moves up to form a barrier between the pharynx and the nasal cavity, so food cannot get into the nasal cavity.

Soft part of the palate
When you swallow, this is the part of the palate that is pushed up, closing the nasal cavity off from the mouth and preventing food from going up the back of the nose.

The conchae

Also known as the turbinate bones, the conchae are bony protrusions into the nasal cavity designed to interrupt the flow of incoming air and cause turbulence. Incoming air bounces around in the nasal cavity picking up heat and moisture, and depositing dust and germs in the mucus that lines the cavity.

The paranasal sinuses

The paranasal sinuses include two frontal cavities, two maxillary cavities, and two anterior ethmoidal sinuses (these last consist of many spaces within the ethmoid bone). There are also two sphenoidal sinuses and the two posterior ethmoidal sinuses, which are positioned too far back in the head to be shown here.

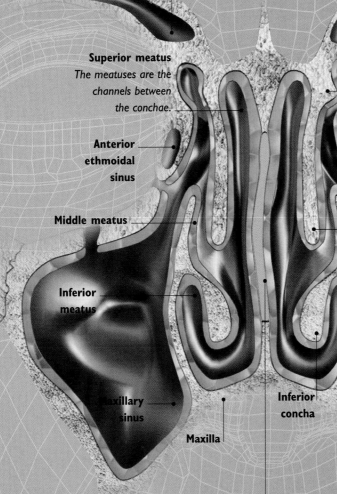

Left and right frontal sinuses

Superior meatus
The meatuses are the channels between the conchae.

Superior concha

Anterior ethmoidal sinus

Middle meatus

Middle concha

Inferior meatus

Maxillary sinus

Inferior concha

Maxilla

The septum *is bony at the back of the nose and composed of cartilage at the front.*

The nasal cavity includes between 10 and 20 million smell receptors, all found within the olfactory region that forms part of the lining of the cavity roof.

Cross-section of the nasal cavity

The nasal cavity and paranasal sinuses are connected by narrow passages, so that air can enter the sinuses from the nasal cavity and mucus manufactured in the sinuses is transported the other way into the nasal cavity, then swallowed.

Smell

Smell is one of the most sensitive and powerful of the primary senses, producing emotional reactions and associations thanks to its unique connections with the brain. It is often underrated and underused by humans.

THE OLFACTORY REGION

Each time you breathe in, air flows around your nasal cavity between the ridges and bumps of the nasal conchae. About 2 per cent of this inhaled air passes over the olfactory region at the top of the nasal cavity that provides your sense of smell (olfactory sense). This olfactory region is rich in sensory receptor cells that sample odour molecules carried on the air; if triggered, they fire off nerve signals to the brain. The olfactory region is unusual in that it connects directly to the brain, and this may account for the emotions, memories and associations that a smell can trigger.

Olfactory receptor cells *are modified nerve cells. A long axon carries nerve signals from the base of each receptor cell into the olfactory bulb and towards the brain.*

Supporting cells *are believed to help clear away unwanted odour molecules that might confuse or swamp the receptor cells. They are covered in tiny hairs called microvilli, which increase their surface area and so makes them more effective.*

The olfactory bulb *is an outgrowth of the brain itself. There are two bulbs – one on each side of the septum that divides the nasal cavity in two.*

Axon

Olfactory bulb

Bone

Mucus glands

Apical knob

Cilia within mucus

The olfactory region within the nasal cavity *is an area of yellowish membrane about the size of a postage stamp.*

The olfactory tract *connects the brain to the olfactory bulb.*

Bone

Superior nasal concha

Olfactory region of the nasal cavity

Nasal cavity

Soft palate

Hard palate

Smelling step-by-step

Olfaction is carried out by specialised receptor cells. These are essentially nerve cells with long hairs called cilia projecting from one end.

1 Odour molecules carried on the air pass over the olfactory region within the nasal cavity.

2 The odour molecules dissolve in the mucus that lines the nasal cavity.

3 The molecules reach receptor cells specialised to respond to their particular odour and bind to receptor molecules on the surface of the receptor cell, triggering a response.

4 The receptor cell sends a nerve signal to the brain.

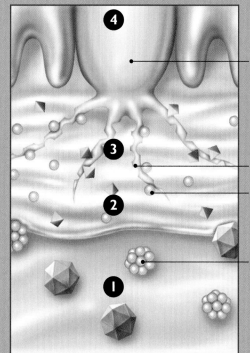

Apical knob: *Each receptor cell is capped with a raised apical knob that projects very slightly through the surface of the olfactory region.*

Cilia: *Sprouting out of each apical knob are around 10 to 20 whip-like filaments called cilia, each 0.0001 mm wide. Cilia increase the surface area to which odour molecules can bind.*

Odour molecule *dissolved in the mucus that lines the nasal cavity.*

Odour molecule *carried along within inhaled air.*

Close-up of a single apical knob
This scanning electron micrograph shows an apical knob – the yellow patch at bottom right – with cilia radiating from its surface.

THE JOURNEY FROM THE NOSE TO THE BRAIN

Axons projecting from the base of each receptor cell join up into nerve bundles. These travel through the bone that separates the nasal cavity from the brain and connect to the olfactory bulb – an outgrowth of the brain itself. From here nerves connect directly to the brain's cortex, where olfactory information is processed. This means that smells are the only sensations to reach the cortex without having to go through the thalamus, a lower brain structure that normally filters and processes incoming information. In addition, the olfactory bulb has direct connections to the brain's limbic system and hippocampus, parts of the brain that are involved in memory and emotion.

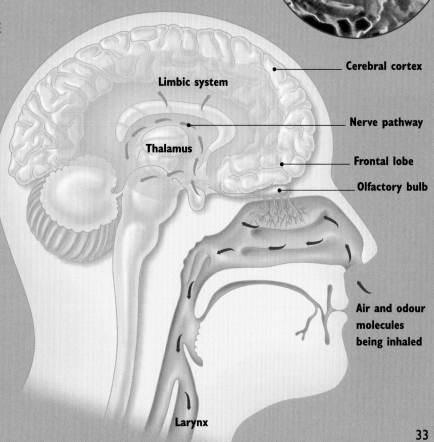

Limbic system

Thalamus

Cerebral cortex

Nerve pathway

Frontal lobe

Olfactory bulb

Air and odour molecules being inhaled

Larynx

The throat and sound production

Leading from the back of the nasal cavity to the top of the trachea and the entrance to the oesophagus, your throat is involved in the key processes of digestion, respiration and speech, or phonation.

The vocal cords are so elastic, they can be stretched by as much as half their length again.

TOUR OF THE THROAT

The throat is made up of the pharynx and the larynx. The pharynx is a 12–14cm (4½–5½in) long muscular tube that leads from the nose and mouth to the top of the oesophagus – the pipe that carries food to the stomach. Near the bottom of the pharynx an opening called the glottis leads to the larynx, a cartilaginous tube that contains the vocal cords and protects the entrance to the trachea, down which air travels to the lungs. The average laryngeal length is 4.5cm (1⅝in) in men but only 3.5cm (1⅜in) in women.

TONSILS AND ADENOIDS

Both tonsils and adenoids are made up of collections of immune cells called lymphocytes that form centres of defence against invading micro-organisms. You'll find the tonsils at the far back and sides of your mouth, within the oropharynx. The adenoids are situated high in the back of the throat behind the nose and the roof of the mouth, in the nasopharynx.

The pharynx *extends in its entirety from the back of the nose to the top of the oesophagus. It has three parts: the nasopharynx, the oropharynx and the laryngopharynx.*

The nasopharynx *runs from the nasal cavity to the soft palate.*

Soft palate

The oropharynx *lies between the soft palate and the glottis.*

Body of the tongue

The glottis *is the gap between the vocal cords.*

The epiglottis *is a hinged piece of cartilage that protects the glottis. When you swallow it swings down to cover the glottis, preventing food or liquid from entering the trachea and lungs.*

Vocal cords

The laryngopharynx *runs from the glottis to the oesophagus.*

The thyroid cartilage *is the largest piece of cartilage in the larynx. It is also called the Adam's apple.*

The larynx – *commonly known as the voice box – is made up of several pieces of cartilage held together with ligaments. It runs from just below the epiglottis to the beginning of the trachea.*

The oesophagus *begins at the base of the neck, just below a ring of cartilage called the crichoid.*

The trachea *starts just below the crichoid cartilage.*

MAKING SOUND

Like any sound production system, the voice box needs three basic components.

An energy source Your breath itself provides the energy for sound production.

An oscillator Your vocal cords and the space between them act as an oscillator. By opening and closing very quickly – up to 250 times per second – the cords set up a series of oscillations in the airstream (in the same fashion as a siren). These determine the basic pitch of the sound.

A resonator Resonation of the vocal cords adds harmonics, without which speech is unintelligible. Your larynx, pharynx and oral and nasal cavities make up your vocal tract, which holds a column of air that acts as a flexible resonator. You can adjust the length, volume, shape and tension of the tract to filter out some of the pitches and harmonics produced by the vocal cords, and amplify and add to others.

Sound bites
The pitch and harmonics produced by your voice box provide the basic vowel sounds of speech, but the addition of consonants, and the way that both vowels and consonants are 'articulated' (shaped and combined), depends on the action of your tongue, palate, lips, cheeks and teeth

THE VOCAL CORDS

The vocal cords are highly elastic ligaments strung across the larynx, with folds or flaps of tissue attached. At the back of the larynx they attach to fingers of mobile cartilage. When you speak, the muscles of your larynx twist and move these cartilages, stretching and flexing the vocal cords in turn. The longer the vocal cords are, the lower their resonant frequency, and the deeper the voice produced. It is because the male vocal cords lengthen at puberty that a boy's voice changes and becomes deeper.

Open and relaxed

Cartilage   Glottis

Epiglottis

Ventricular fold

Vocal cord, also known as a vocal fold.

Closed and taut

During normal breathing the vocal cords are relaxed and open. When you speak or sing, they are pulled more or less taut.

The ventricular folds are flaps of tissue that close off the glottis when you swallow and protect the vocal cords. They are also called the false vocal cords.

A day in the life of your ears, nose and throat

Your ears, nose and throat are highly responsive to changes in both the external and internal environment. Conscious control, involuntary reflexes and chemical messengers combine to fine-tune their day-to-day functioning.

HOME AND AWAY

Your ears, nose and throat are controlled by a combination of nerve signals from the brain and local control mechanisms. The ear, for example, can protect itself against damage from loud noises with the help of feedback from the brain, while the mucous lining of the sinuses responds to signals from local immune tissues. Your ears, nose and throat also help to control other systems of your body, such as head orientation and facial muscle action.

08: 00 Nasal intelligence

As you head for the kitchen for breakfast you realise that your partner has the coffee on already – your nostrils flare to capture more of the rich aroma and suddenly you remember the Parisian café where you breakfasted as a student. Your reverie is interrupted by a less pleasant smell: as you become aware that the toast is burning, signals are sent to the facial muscles around your nose, stimulating them to contract and producing a wrinkling of the nose. This narrows the nostrils and prevents more odour molecules from getting in.

8:45 Under pressure

On your journey to work he train enters a tunnel. This causes the air pressure around you to increase, while the air in your middle ear is still at the same pressure as before. This produces a feeling of discomfort, and prevents the accurate transmission of sound waves through the ossicles, so that everything sounds dulled. You swallow, causing your larynx to rise and your pharynx to contract. This opens the end of the eustachian tube, letting air into your middle ear, equalising the pressure and enabling you to hear normally again.

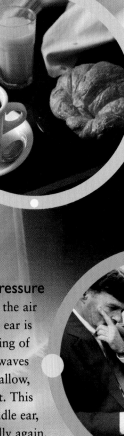

Taking time out
Playing with your sense of balance on the rides at a fair or theme park can be fun. A rollercoaster ride sends the otoliths within the vestibule of your inner ear into freefall, as your head is pulled back and forth by the fierce tug of gravity.

22:00 Time to relax – and rest

The day is drawing to a close and all you want to do is unwind before going to bed. You run a deep bath, into which you pour some bath lotion and a few drops of your favourite aromatherapy oil. As you lie back and take the first of a series of slow, relaxing breaths, the bath oil begins to work its magic. Soothing vapours are gently sucked into your nasal cavity, where their aroma is picked up by sensory receptor cells in the olfactory region on the roof of the nasal cavity. From here, nerve signals to the olfactory bulb in the brain trigger feelings of peace, pleasure and letting go – a fitting end to the day.

17:30 Keeping your balance

You head for the sports centre after work and as you lunge up, down, forward and sideways, it is your sense of balance that saves you from falling flat on your face. Tiny cilia attached to hair cells within the semicircular canals and vestibule of your inner ear move in the same direction as your head. The resulting nerve signals allow you to maintain a precise awareness of the speed and angle of your head – key knowledge when it comes to controlling the movement of your body.

11:30 Volume control

There's a lot of drilling at a building site next to the office, which sends blasts of very loud sound waves into your ear, causing large movements of the hairs in your ear's cochlea. A nerve signal races towards your brainstem (where the brain meets the spinal cord) and triggers a reflex feedback signal to the muscles attached to your ossicles within the middle ear. The muscles contract, damping the excessive and potentially damaging vibrations of the ossicles and thereby also protecting your cochlear receptor hairs. At the same time, another reflex nerve signal from the brainstem activates your neck muscles, turning your head so you face the source of the sound.

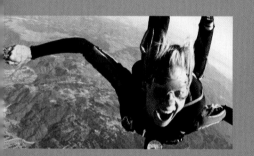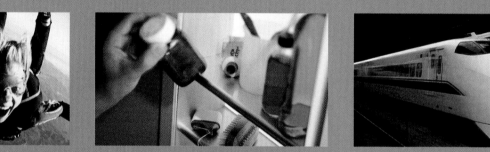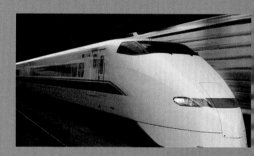

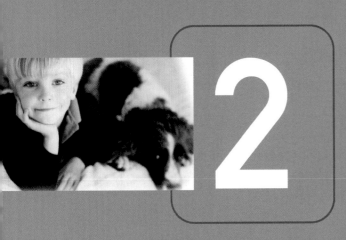

2

Keeping your ears, nose and throat healthy

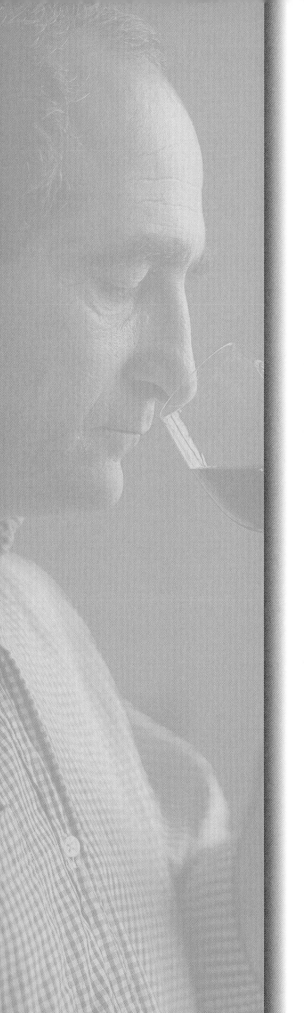

CARING FOR THE EARS, NOSE AND THROAT

The ears, nose and throat are in constant contact with outside stimuli and much of the time they function without us being aware of them, but problems in one area may impact on the others.

 41 *Understanding how your ears, nose and throat work, and the relationship between them, is the first step to good health.*

 44 *Simple good habits in your daily life can help to achieve a lifetime of good health for your ears, nose and throat.*

 46 *The senses of hearing, smell and taste change as we age. Knowing the changes to expect enables you to seek help early for a problem.*

 51 *Niggling symptoms affect the ears, nose and throat often, so it is important to know when to ignore and when to treat them.*

 54 *Understanding how infections of the ears, nose and throat are spread will enable you to treat them swiftly and effectively.*

 55 *Both pharmacists and complementary therapists have a wealth of remedies to treat common ENT ailments.*

 59 *Being a wise traveller can help you to avoid motion sickness and other potential problems of the ears, nose and throat.*

Understanding your ENT

Learning how your ears, nose and throat function both independently from one another and how they are related gives you the knowledge you need to sense when your ENT health might be changing for the worse.

YOUR EARS AND HEARING

Of the five senses, hearing probably does the most in helping you to communicate with the world around you. Your ears are simply amazing, allowing you to enjoy a Beethoven recital, join in a conversation or hear a police siren. If your ears are functioning correctly, this usually happens unconsciously.

It is only when you concentrate on a specific sound that you become aware of using your sense of hearing. Your ears not only perceive sounds of very low and very high pitch but are also able to detect varying intensities of sound. The sounds that you hear are a result of many single frequencies being integrated into a tone by your brain.

We all take our hearing for granted and, quite often, hearing loss can go undetected for some time, particularly if it is gradual or in only one ear. If you are concerned about the quality of your hearing, there are several questions you can ask yourself to ascertain whether or not you might have a problem (see page 52).

Dual signals

Most sounds can be distinguished perfectly well with one ear alone. The task of pinpointing where a sound comes from, however, is dependent on both ears. The brain interprets the subtle differences in data from each ear and combines them. Pattern recognition can tell us whose voice we are hearing or what car is arriving. The human ear is so specialised that not only can we recognise the similarities between sounds so that words are heard, but we can also detect enough to know exactly who is speaking.

Sound overload
Your ears have to detect thousands of different sounds every day, and then pass on this information to your brain which interprets what those sounds are, and prepares your body for a response.

41

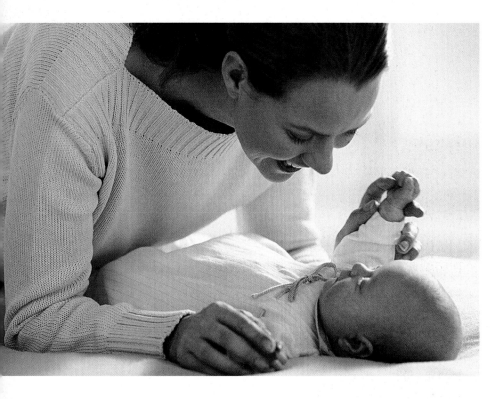

Unique scent
In one study, babies as young as six weeks correctly identified their own mother's teeshirt by scent.

KEEPING YOUR BALANCE

Staying upright is governed by your inner ear. It responds to your head's movement and position relative to gravity, and triggers a response in the brain to restore the equilibrium. The inner ear needs help, however, and balance relies to a considerable extent on the eyes as well. They send similar messages to the brain, based on movement. Your sense of balance is challenged when the messages from the inner ear and the eyes differ – often during times of speed and motion, such as on a rollercoaster.

A NORMAL NOSE

You rely on your sense of smell for more information about your surroundings than you probably realise. It is important in all animal behaviour, for identification of food, mates and predators. For humans, it also provides sensual pleasure, as well as warning of dangers such as spoiled food and escaping gas.

Are you led by your nose?

Perfume companies try to tell us that wearing their products will instantly make us more sexually attractive. However, studies have indicated that we have our own smell-signalling system. Chemicals called pheromones may partly govern our sexual identification and behaviour.

In humans, the most important odour-producing organ is the skin, whose apocrine glands produce substances detectable only by the human nose. However, there is another scent detection system, located on the nasal septum, that may also detect these chemicals.

Scientists have demonstrated that by six weeks of age babies can differentiate their own mother's smell. In addition, it has been observed since the 1960s that, under the influence of pheromones, women living in the same house tend to have periods at around the same time of month. Young adults can distinguish their own scent from others and can also differentiate male from female body odour on clothing.

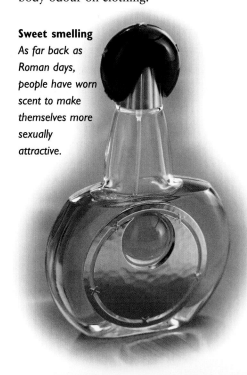

Sweet smelling
As far back as Roman days, people have worn scent to make themselves more sexually attractive.

THE THROAT

Your throat contains two important areas of immune cells called the tonsils and adenoids. In children these are important at fighting off respiratory tract and lung infections, but they can become so enlarged that they interfere with the functioning of the ears, nose and throat. Following adolescence they become redundant and shrink and few adults are aware of their presence.

At the base of your throat lies the larynx – yet another part of your ears, nose and throat involved in communication. When functioning poorly, the larynx displays signs of hoarseness or loss of voice, which you will experience as a 'sore' throat.

INTERRELATED SYSTEMS

Your ears, nose and throat are closely related both in terms of structure and function. A problem in any one of these organs can spread to or produce symptoms in another. Not only are the three connected, they all produce warm fluid – a perfect medium for bacteria and viruses to multiply.

An infection in the nose or throat can easily spread to the ears or to the paranasal sinuses, which become blocked by fluid. An ear infection may cause balance problems, while enlarged adenoids can block the eustachian tube, causing pain in the ear and the nose, making breathing difficult. Conversely, an obstruction in the nasal space can block ears.

A blocked eustachian tube can also arise during a bad cold or hay fever and produce pain on swallowing and fluid in the middle ear.

Colds and hay fever can produce symptoms in all these organs, either all at once or one after another.

WELL CONNECTED

The interrelationship of your ears, nose and throat explains why discomfort or infection in one part of the system may easily spread to another. All are connected in more ways than one, with some perhaps surprising parts of the ENT system directly joined. The labels below identify the most important connections.

NOSE – SINUSES
The nose is connected to the paranasal sinuses, which drain fluid into the nose.

NASAL CAVITY – PHARYNX
The nasal cavity is connected to the nasopharynx.

EARS – THROAT
The ears are connected directly with the throat by the eustachian tube, which opens and closes to allow air to enter the middle ear, keeping it at atmospheric pressure.

EARS – THROAT
The eustachian tube also carries catarrh produced in the middle ear to the throat, where it can be swallowed.

THROAT – OESOPHAGUS
The throat connects the mouth and oesophagus. During swallowing food is directed down the oesophagus.

THROAT – WINDPIPE
The throat is connected to the windpipe where air passes on its way to and from the lungs.

The ears, nose and throat in daily life

Your ears, nose and throat are constantly bombarded by pollutants, viruses, bacteria, pollen, alcohol, noise, air pressure …the list is endless. How your body reacts to irritants can have an effect on your day-to-day activities and well-being.

When they are working well, you are likely to be almost unaware of your ears, nose and throat. Several everyday situations have an impact on them, however. Knowing when they might be compromised enables you to take sensible precautions to preserve your health.

PREVENT EAR INFECTIONS

Acute earache is usually the result of an infection in the inner ear, most often caused by the bacteria or viruses from a cold or flu travelling along the eustachian tube and settling there. The infection stimulates an increase in secretion from the mucous membrane but, often, the eustachian tube is so inflamed by the infection that the fluids are unable to drain out. The structure of the eustachian tube in children allows viruses and bacteria to reach the middle ear much more frequently, with a greater risk of infection. The adenoids are relatively larger in children than in adults and can press on the opening to the eustachian tube, which can prevent catarrh from draining out of the middle ear and increase the risk of an ear infection.

Poorly functioning eustachian tubes can cause the sensation of muffled hearing and pain. In severe cases the eardrum may perforate.

HOW TO BLOW YOUR NOSE

Believe it or not, there is a right way and a wrong way to blow your nose. If you apply too much pressure you risk forcing harmful bacteria into your sinus cavities or ears or even

Depressurise
The rapid drop in pressure during a sky dive presents serious risk to the ears – during a jump it is vital to equalise the pressure in your ears to prevent damage.

rupturing an eardrum. The best advice is to blow one nostril at a time, while pressing gently on the other one. Blow frequently to prevent mucus build up and use a tissue. A dab of petroleum jelly around the nostrils may help to prevent soreness.

CHANGING PRESSURE

Air is usually able to pass freely into the middle ear to maintain atmospheric pressure. Under certain circumstances, however, your ears are affected by a change in pressure, and you might find yourself suffering from barotrauma, or pressure damage. To protect yourself:

As many as 85 per cent of infections of the middle ear are experienced by the under 12s.

0-5 YEARS

Help your child to avoid infection

Breastfeeding offers some immunity to infections; in addition, the action of breastfeeding – a strong suck followed by a swallow – inhibits the flow of milk into the eustachian tube. Bottles, by contrast, can provoke infection as milk can pool and flow into the eustachian tube, where it provides a perfect breeding ground for bacteria. Some doctors believe that sucking a dummy promotes the flow of fluids from a baby's mouth and into the eustachian tube and do not recommend it. Teaching children to blow their nose as young as possible might prevent some episodes of ear infection by clearing catarrh from the nasal cavity and preventing it from entering the middle ear.

- Be alert to the risks of barotrauma when flying (see page 62).
- Know the risks of any hobbies you undertake, such as diving or bungee jumping.
- Take time to become acclimatised to altitude before exerting yourself.

Nosebleeds, too, can be caused by a rapid change in air pressure and by exposure to high altitude.

TURN IT DOWN!

Sensorineural hearing loss – that caused by noise – is preventable. Your ears are not designed to listen to loud noise: if noise is loud enough and lasts for long enough, it will damage your hearing. As exposure time increases, more and more nerve endings in the

inner ear are destroyed and they cannot regenerate. If you have grown used to a loud noise it has probably already damaged your ears, and no treatment will help (see page 80).

A GOOD NIGHT'S SLEEP

Unfortunately, you are not the only person who may be troubled by a problem with your ears, nose or throat. Up to 25 per cent of the population snore, disturbing not only their own sleep, but also that of the people they live with. Snoring can be a serious social and medical problem.

Snoring occurs when the tongue and soft palate collapse during sleep, causing a blockage in the air passage which prevents the sleeper from breathing normally. The sound

produced is made by the collapsed parts of the mouth vibrating and striking each other during breathing. Snoring is most common in children and in people over forty years old, and can be the result of many factors including swollen adenoids, alcohol, sleeping tablets, being overweight and smoking. You can also snore if your nose is blocked by a cold, hay fever or nasal polyps.

Countless methods have been devised in an attempt to cure snoring, and range from the age-old method of sewing a ball into the back of the pyjamas to nasal sprays and headgear that repositions the jaw. It is true that such inventions are likely to stop you from snoring – but only by keeping you awake.

CHANGES FOR A SNORE-FREE NIGHT

Some simple lifestyle changes can have a great impact on your quality of sleep. None of the methods here need medical help, or require you to sleep in discomfort. Try them out and see which works for you, so that you and the people around you get a better night's sleep.

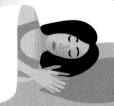

Get fit *By getting more exercise and losing a few excess pounds, not only will you improve muscle tone, but you will also lose bulky neck tissue which causes snoring by narrowing the airways.*

Be habitual *Establish regular sleeping patterns and go to bed at the same time each night. Sleep deprivation can be a cause of snoring.*

Eating and drinking *Don't eat for three hours before sleeping – saliva and mucus production can interfere with breathing – and don't drink alcohol for four hours as alcohol can over-relax the muscles. Drink a glass of warm milk before turning in, as milk contains an amino acid that induces sleep.*

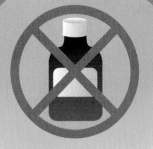

Sleep naturally *Do not take sleeping pills or tranquillisers before going to bed as they relax the muscles too much.*

The right position *Go to sleep on your side rather than on your back, and prop your head up four inches with pillows.*

How your ENT change with age

As our bodies mature, the performance of our ears, nose and throat changes. Generally it deteriorates with age, but certain stages of life, such as illness or pregnancy, can have a profound effect on functioning.

HOW HEARING CHANGES

Periods of temporary hearing loss are common, particularly associated with colds and other infections. Some degree of hearing loss, however, is a normal part of the ageing process. Unfortunately, this is a permanent condition, but there are increasing numbers of aids that can be used to assist with hearing.

Age-related hearing loss

Permanent, age-related hearing loss tends to occur in families. Referred to as presbyacusis, this is usually associated with a genetic predisposition rather than noise trauma, although persistent exposure to loud noise also causes hearing loss

As hearing matures

At birth, our ears are sensitive to wavelengths between 40 and 20,000Hz. A child can often distinguish sounds from 20Hz (lowest note on an organ) to 20,000Hz, and hearing stays within these frequencies in adulthood. As we age, it becomes less acute.

(see page 80). Generally, as age increases, so too does loss of hearing. It begins with high-frequency sounds such as speech, particularly high-frequency consonants such as 't', 'p', 'k' and 'f'. Such hearing loss can often go undetected for quite some time because the onset is usually gradual: most experts agree that it usually begins during our 50s, although some suggest it starts as early as the 30s.

In addition to losing the ability to hear high-frequency sounds, the ability to detect quiet sounds starts to diminish as we age. Some experts quantify hearing loss as mild, severe and profound depending on a person's inability to distinguish sounds at particular levels. Mild hearing loss is the inability to hear 25–30dB, for example above the background hum of a quiet office; severe loss is the inability to hear 40–60dB, the level of normal speech; and a person who cannot hear 90dB, for example a loud radio, has profound hearing loss.

How is sound measured?

There are two ways of measuring sound. Sounds are produced by the vibration of particles in the air which travel as sound waves. The distance between each peak of sound energy is called a wavelength, measured in cycles per second (Hertz or Hz). This so-called frequency determines the sound's pitch. The other measure is the sound's pressure level, a measure of its intensity, which is calibrated in decibels (dB, see page 81).

ASK THE EXPERT

About a quarter of people aged 65–75 years old and half of those over 75 suffer from some degree of hearing loss. There are only 16,000 fine-hair sound-detector cells in the average cochlea, and most people will have lost about one-third of them by the time they are 65. These cells are irreplaceable.

Conductive hearing loss

It is not uncommon, either during childhood or adulthood, to experience a loss of hearing owing to a blockage which prevents sound from entering the inner ear. Such episodes of hearing loss are often temporary, and can usually be treated easily, fully restoring hearing to normal. As we age, one of the more frequent reasons for this type of hearing loss is the build-up of earwax. Earwax becomes drier as we get older, and is also more easily compacted. It is, however, a simple exercise in the GP's surgery to have it removed (see pages 116–17).

Keeping tuned in

In so-called assistive listening devices, sound is amplified and delivered via headphones and earphones to enable you to hear a stereo, a telephone (either with an amplified handset or an extra ear piece), television or radio.

Alarm calls

The usual sound signal in door bells, alarm clocks, baby alarms and smoke detectors can be changed to a flashing light or vibration system. Extensions or remote units can be sited in other rooms or simply moved around the house so that a light flashes when supper is ready, for example. Alarm clocks can be fixed to vibration systems that wake you in bed.

DEVICES TO HELP WITH HEARING LOSS

Daily life is full of situations that can be frustrating for those with a degree of hearing loss and also those close to them: difficulty speaking on the telephone, for example, or having the television or radio turned up very loud.

Since many causes of adult hearing loss are untreatable, the major tasks of the doctor, audiologist and hearing therapist are to prevent further hearing loss if possible and rehabilitate remaining useful hearing. If you suspect that your hearing is not as acute as it once was, don't delay. The sooner you are seen the better: some aids take a little getting used to.

A wide range of equipment is available to aid hearing and communication, all of which may improve the quality of a person's life.

In your ear

There is a vast array of hearing aids suitable for most people with various causes of hearing loss. They act as an amplifier and improve the hearing that you have left: they cannot replace lost hearing. It can take weeks, if not months, to adjust to the amplified sounds, particularly in those who have been deaf for some time. Aids can be worn on the body, behind the ear and in the ear, and the most suitable type will depend on the cause and extent of an individual's hearing loss.

Staying in touch

A wide variety of state-of-the-art communication equipment is available. Devices such as text-telephones and computerised notepads allow understanding of the spoken language, enable two-way communication without a human interpreter, improve reading skills and help with learning sign languages.

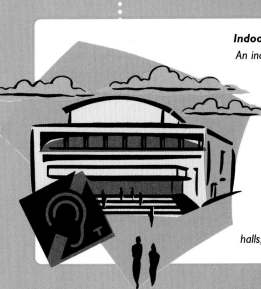

Indoor environments

An induction loop fitted into a building converts sound signals into electrical impulses through a wire. The current sets up a magnetic field in the wire that can be picked up by a hearing aid switched to the correct setting. These sounds are unaffected by distance or background noise, so are extremely useful in public places such as conference rooms, theatres, concert halls, ticket offices and doctors' surgeries.

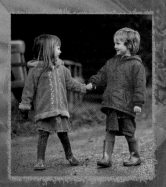

SCENTS IN THE RISE
A child's sense of smell matures from birth and is as acute as a young adult's by around the age of eight.

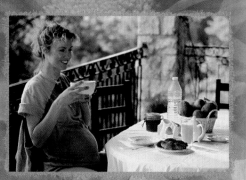

TESTING TIMES
Pregnancy is often a time of heightened sensitivity, with many stronger odours provoking nausea and vomiting.

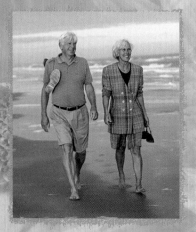

THE DECLINE OF ADULTHOOD
The sense of smell certainly declines as we grow older, although the age at which this begins is debated.

THE CHANGING SENSE OF SMELL

Some people have a keener sense of smell than others, but we all experience a weakness or loss of smell – and often of the intertwined sense of taste with it – at some point during our lives.

For the most part, we tend to rely on our eyes and ears rather than our sense of smell to determine our social behaviour. From an evolutionary point of view this is an advanced state – dogs, for example, 'follow their noses' for food, territory, finding family and mating. Ants follow a complex system of social behaviour patterns related to their sense of smell. Yet mothers can recognise their own baby from smell alone in the same way that a newborn infant locates its mother's nipple by smell. Our ways of finding mates are also partially dependent on invisible smell signals from pheromones (see page 42).

A heightened sense of smell

Some people develop aversions to certain smells. This is by far most common in pregnancy and is closely bound up with the nausea and vomiting of early pregnancy. During this time the placenta produces increasing amounts of oestrogen to keep the fetus healthy. A side effect of this is that women can detect volatile chemicals in, for example, coffee, tea, tobacco, petroleum products, perfume and some foods, and find them intolerably strong. Pregnant women often say that it is a smell that triggers their vomiting. It also seems that women who are born infertile, if helped to conceive, are less likely to suffer from morning

sickness. Research is on-going to prove the exact links between oestrogen and the sense of smell.

The taste-smell connection

Your senses of smell and taste are very closely linked. Both depend on the recognition of chemical molecules from substances around you, and which stimulate specialised nerve cells in your nose, mouth and throat. These nerve cells produce electrical impulses, which are taken to parts of the brain where smells and tastes are recognised. As many as 10,000 taste buds are located on the upper surface of your tongue, but these can only distinguish between sweet, sour, bitter and salt stimuli. Other factors such as texture and temperature play a part in recognising a particular 'taste', but more important are the smell receptors high in the nasal cavity. Some flavours rely more on smell than taste for their identification. These include chocolate and coffee: if you hold your nose while you eat chocolate, all you will be able to tell is whether it is sweet or bitter.

A weakened sense of smell

Your sense of smell declines in old age. This is in keeping with the general loss of brain function that occurs with ageing. The olfactory bulb – which carries smell from the odour detectors in the nasal cavity to the brain – gets smaller as we age and the nerve cells in the nose that detect smells become thinner and more spread out, so are less effective. This can be dangerous as it may lead

Up to one in 10 people complain of problems with taste and smell at some time in their lives.

to a reduced ability to detect dangerous smells such as gas, or food that has gone off.

A few people are born with a poor sense of smell, but the problem is usually an acquired one. You may lose your sense of smell temporarily if you have a blocked nose, for example, or permanently after a serious head injury. Localised nasal problems, such as polyps or a deviated nasal septum, can also cause a loss of the sense of smell. Allergies can thicken the membrane lining the nose and thereby reduce smell acuity. Recent research has pointed to the loss of the sense of smell being an early sign of Alzheimer's disease, a condition which affects more women than men (see page 110). There have also been reported instances of temporary desensitisation to smells. Workers in chocolate factories, for example, are

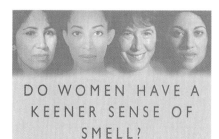

DO WOMEN HAVE A KEENER SENSE OF SMELL?

Women have a more sensitive and wider ranging sense of smell than men or children. This is thought to be because oestrogen, the female hormone, increases the action of the olfactory nerve cells. Women are generally much more sensitive to the odour of musk, similar to the male hormone testosterone, than men, who are relatively insensitive. The level of a woman's sensitivity to this smell varies according to the stage in her menstrual cycle, again probably related to the amount of oestrogen circulating. Women on the pill (who do not ovulate), women whose ovaries have been removed and post-menopausal women have a less acute sense of smell and in some cases complain that they have completely lost their sense of smell.

reputed not to smell the chocolate after a while. However, the chocolate smells as strong to someone returning after a week's holiday as it does to a newcomer to the factory.

Professional noses

Although some people do have a better sense of smell than others, most who consider themselves good 'noses' agree that this is primarily a matter of being aware of smells, and of practising noticing the distinctions between them.

YOUR CHANGING VOICE

From the high-pitched cry of a newborn baby to the deep bass tones of the adult man, our voices change as we age. Although these changes are most dramatic in adolescent males, all our voices evolve at almost every stage of life.

Factors that influence our voices as we age include: growth, which affects vocal cord length; the development of muscles in the neck; the changing structure of the tissues of the vocal cords; and the increasing boniness of cartilage of the larynx.

A child's voice

At birth, the vocal cords which vibrate to produce sound, are about 2mm long. Throughout childhood these grow about 0.7mm each year in boys and 0.4mm a year in girls. In spite of their smaller vocal cords and smaller lungs, however, children can produce sounds as loud as adults because they make sounds of a higher frequency. They also have a higher lung pressure that allows them to work harder than adults to produce sound.

> *Human speech frequencies vary between 50 and 4000Hz.*

Changes at adolescence

Men and women have different voice pitches and this is directly related to the size of the larynx.

Testosterone production in boys, from puberty onwards, causes their larynx to lengthen, and thickens the vocal cords. This produces different pitches and harmonics. Initially, boys may alternate between their pre-pubertal high-pitched voice and a deeper tone, sometimes producing a mix of the two as the boy becomes accustomed to the change, but gradually the deeper voice stabilises.

The changes in girls' voices are less dramatic, but they do become increasingly breathless and husky, and lower in frequency.

Adulthood

The loudness and quality of your voice generally stabilises during the mid-life years. However, the larynx slowly descends and thickens with age. A man's voice continues to deepen as he grows older, though after about 70 its pitch goes up again slightly due to falling testosterone levels, and it can sound thinner and more reedy. A woman's voice, by contrast, becomes deeper and more husky. By the time men and women reach their 90s, they sound much the same; also, older people may speak more slowly and their voices can sound more tremulous.

Combining voices
Voice pitch varies from male to female and with age. A successful singing ensemble exploits these differences.

What is a voiceprint?

Some experts argue that we each have an individual 'voiceprint'. Every person's vocal cords process sounds slightly differently, and the way each person produces sound – the use of the tongue, mouth, lips, and so on – also differs. The combination of these factors makes it unlikely that two voices would be exactly alike. The voiceprint is a trace measured on a machine called a spectrograph registering how high and low a voice is and its Hz frequency. Although critics argue against the accuracy of voiceprints, they have been used in criminal investigations in the USA.

ASK THE EXPERT

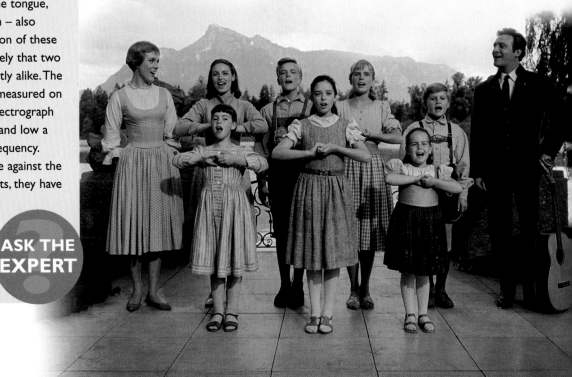

Looking out for symptoms

You will experience symptoms from your ears, nose and throat fairly frequently. As with other body systems, the important thing is knowing how to distinguish between what is serious and what is trivial.

Recognising the various symptoms that can indicate an ear, nose or throat problem will help you to decide on your best course of action. If you are not sure whether your symptoms necessitate a visit to the doctor, phone the practice nurse for advice. Persistent symptoms, even if they appear trivial, should prompt a visit to the doctor.

NOSEBLEEDS

A nosebleed in a child with a cold is not usually of concern, although the nasal lining may be likely to bleed again if the nose is blown too enthusiastically. Encourage frequent light nose blowing (see page 44). Nosebleeds at other times may run in the family and are usually no cause for concern: children grow out of them by their teens. However, consult a doctor if a child with a nosebleed:
• is pale, sweaty and unresponsive;
• has lost a lot of blood;
• has had a blow to the nose;
• is vomiting blood.
Nosebleeds in adults can be an indication of something more serious such as high blood pressure. A nosebleed that doesn't stop after 15 minutes is a medical emergency.

SINUS PAIN

Sometimes it is difficult to distinguish between an ordinary headache and one caused by blocked or infected sinuses. If the answer to any of these questions is yes, the pain may be caused by sinus disease and you should see your doctor.

• Do you feel the pain mainly in your face and forehead?
• Does the pain worsen when you bend over?
• Have you recently had a runny nose and high temperature?
• Do you have a discoloured or blood-stained nasal discharge?

EARACHE

Earache is much more common in young children. If your baby or toddler is screaming and pulling their ears, suspect a middle ear infection (acute otitis media). These symptoms may also be associated with a discharge of pus, and sometimes blood, if the eardrum has perforated. Your child should see a doctor who will prescribe antibiotics.

In adults, too, earache may signify a middle ear infection. If it is accompanied by a blocked sensation in the ear, it may be due to pressure damage or eustachian tube malfunction. Pain that is worse if you pull on your outer ear may be due to a boil in the ear canal or possibly an infection of the skin of the ear canal.

Discharge from the ear

In children and adults this is commonly associated with an infection of the outer ear canal, which might also accompany a sore, itchy and painful ear, or a perforated eardrum. Causes may include swimmer's ear, eczema, psoriasis or (especially in children) a foreign body in the ear.

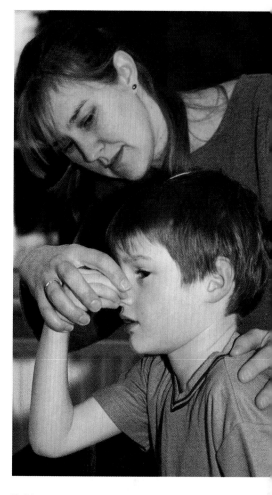

Hold your nose
A person with a nosebleed should sit with the head upright and pinch both nostrils together for at least 15 minutes. The method of tipping the head back simply allows blood to trickle down the throat, causing coughing.

Middle ear infection

An infection may also cause discharge if the eardrum develops a hole so that pus and blood escape. This usually relieves the severe pain. A clear or blood-stained discharge from the ear or nose after an injury needs emergency medical treatment.

COLDS

At least 200 viruses are known to cause the common cold, and you are more likely to succumb in the

ASSESSING LOSS OF HEARING

If you have any concerns about your ability to hear, ask yourself these questions to decide whether to see the doctor.

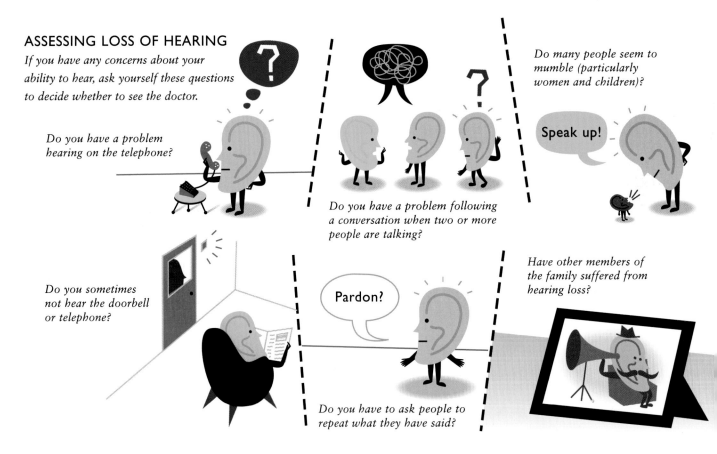

Do you have a problem hearing on the telephone?

Do you have a problem following a conversation when two or more people are talking?

Do many people seem to mumble (particularly women and children)?

Speak up!

Do you sometimes not hear the doorbell or telephone?

Pardon?

Have other members of the family suffered from hearing loss?

Do you have to ask people to repeat what they have said?

---

autumn or winter. The symptoms of sneezing, blocked and runny nose, sore throat and feverishness develop between 12 hours and 3 days after catching the infection. Colds are minor self-limiting illnesses lasting a few days only, unless you develop complications, which are more likely in children and older people. Children commonly develop ear infections after a cold; adults may have sinusitis or a chest infection.

Blocked or runny nose

The lining membrane of your nose can swell and produce fluid for a number of reasons. The most common by far is a virus infection, or common cold. A blocked nose may also be caused by an anatomical distortion of the nose after a fracture or by nasal polyps. If you are also suffering an itchy nose and eyes then

the likely cause is allergy. If the symptoms are seasonal, this may be an allergy to pollen, moulds or spores and is termed seasonal rhinitis; if it is persistent, it is likely to be due to the house-dust mite.

Sneezing

This is the nose's defence mechanism to try to expel unwanted substances. It can be caused by an allergy, irritant or infection.

SORE THROAT

Soreness in the throat may be due to exposure to either pollutants or irritants such as cigarette smoke. In addition, shouting and other voice stressors can cause a sore throat (see page 68).

Soreness of the throat along with a fever and aches and pains may indicate tonsillitis. Sore throat, fever

and swollen glands in your neck, armpits or groins could indicate glandular fever. You should visit the doctor in both cases.

IT'S NOT TRUE!

'Nasal discharge tells you what's wrong'

Some people believe that clear nasal discharge indicates a viral infection while yellow/green discharge means a bacterial infection. The colour of the discharge, however, simply reflects the number of white blood cells fighting off the infection. A yellowish discharge means that white blood cell production is in full swing.

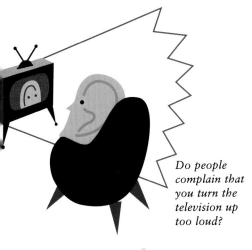

Do people complain that you turn the television up too loud?

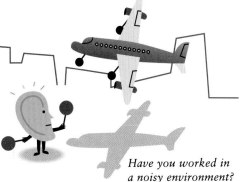

Have you worked in a noisy environment?

Certain prescription drugs such as some antibiotics can cause a drop in the white blood cell count, which may provoke a sore throat.

Hoarseness, loss of voice

Hoarseness is a change in quality or volume of your voice caused by alteration in your vocal cords which can swell or develop nodules from overuse. This can be due to a viral infection (common cold, laryngitis), specific occupations such as singing or teaching, or pollutants and irritants like cigarette smoke.

If your voice has changed slowly at the same time as your skin and hair have become dry, or you feel excessively tired, you may have an underactive thyroid gland. In smokers, a hoarse voice can be a symptom of a more serious problem such as throat or lung cancer.

Difficulty swallowing

Accompanied with a sore throat, a swallowing problem may be caused by an object lodged in your throat. If you feel that food gets stuck high up in your gullet, you may have acid reflux. This can also cause a recurrent cough and sore throat. Anxiety can cause the sensation of a lump in the throat, but in such cases swallowing is normal.

HEARING PROBLEMS

Up to one in 1000 newborn babies is profoundly deaf and nearly one in 20 has significant hearing impairment. Screening tests are available and babies benefit from early intervention. Tell your health visitor or doctor if, from your baby's reactions to noise, you suspect a hearing deficiency.

Problems in older children can be harder to pinpoint as some children seem to 'screen out' adults deliberately, but a child who needs the television turned up louder than normal should probably be checked out. Hearing problems can also cause under-performance at school, so if your child's performance seems to have tailed off, suspect hearing difficulties. Possible causes for this are inherited forms of deafness, an infection such as rubella, or glue ear.

In adults, hearing loss can affect all sounds or just some frequencies, and may be sudden or gradual. There may be a family history of deafness. Other possibilities are overexposure to loud noise, or wax build-up in the outer ear canal. Half of all over-70s have some degree of age-related hearing loss and people should discuss coping strategies with their doctor and family sooner rather than later (see page 47).

(see page 47).

Does milk cause mucus production?

TALKING POINT

Despite many scientific trials on the subject, contrary medical opinions, and anecdotal evidence, there has been no scientific evidence to link mucus production with milk. Many people find that drinking milk leaves a soft filmy coating in the mouth and throat, but this substance should not be confused with mucus. A recent study in Australia found that the 'mucus effect' of cow's milk is most likely just the milk itself, probably combined with slightly increased saliva levels, and not an increase in mucus production. An inability to tolerate milk products is likely to be lactose intolerance, or in rare cases milk allergy.

Sudden hearing loss in one ear only is an emergency as it can result in permanent hearing loss: seek urgent medical help. The most common cause for this is a viral infection but occasionally a benign tumour of the auditory nerve is diagnosed.

Tinnitus

Tinnitus sufferers hear persistent noises in the ear, indicating damage to the middle or inner ear. The noises may be high or low in pitch, they may be buzzing or sibilant, and they can continue night and day. Possible causes include Ménière's disease, exposure to loud noise, and certain medication, such as aspirin, taken in high doses, but in many cases there is no identifiable cause.

How infections are spread

Infections of the ears, nose and throat are common, partly because these organs are the main entrance to the body through which all food, fluid and air passes. As such, they offer free entry to a host of bacteria and viruses too.

Infectious diseases are caused by microorganisms that invade your body. They cause inflammation and immune responses that then produce symptoms of a particular illness.

VIRUSES

Most ear, nose and throat infections are caused by viruses, some others by bacteria, and relatively few by fungi or parasites. Viruses can only grow or divide in living cells. More than 200 different viruses can cause the common cold.

Airborne disease

Viruses pass from person to person in droplets of mucus produced by an already infected person. The virus particles are expelled by coughing or sneezing and inhaled to impact on the mucous membrane of the recipient. Even when a handkerchief is used, the droplet range for a sneeze can be several feet. One study found that, in the infectious stage of a cold, more than 6000 viable droplets were produced every hour, and these can remain airborne for up to 10 minutes.

Contact contamination

Cold viruses can also live for some hours on skin and other surfaces, so picking up a child, handing someone a plate or the TV remote control, or sharing a towel can all spread the infection, as can shaking a contaminated hand. If you have a cold, be sure to wash your hands often to avoid spreading it to others.

WHO GETS INFECTIONS?

It is also important to remember that an individual's chances of catching a cold depend on several factors:
- The length of exposure: 8 hours a day in close contact with an infected person increases the risk.
- Health status: someone whose immunity is compromised is more likely to catch a cold, so the old and young are especially at risk.

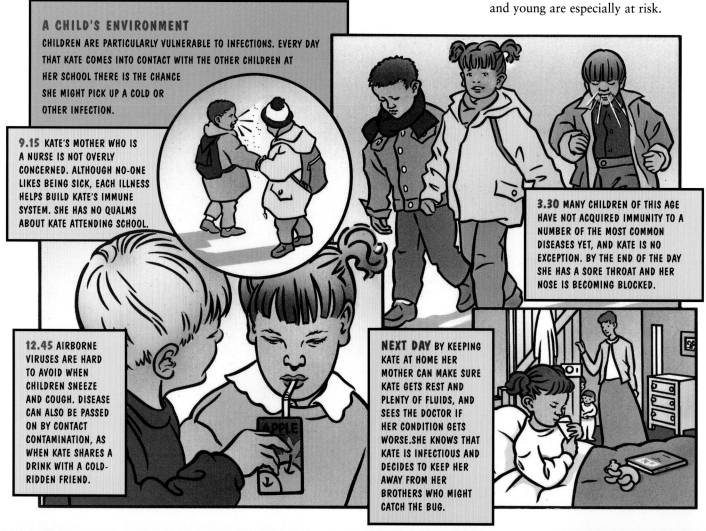

A CHILD'S ENVIRONMENT
CHILDREN ARE PARTICULARLY VULNERABLE TO INFECTIONS. EVERY DAY THAT KATE COMES INTO CONTACT WITH THE OTHER CHILDREN AT HER SCHOOL THERE IS THE CHANCE SHE MIGHT PICK UP A COLD OR OTHER INFECTION.

9.15 KATE'S MOTHER WHO IS A NURSE IS NOT OVERLY CONCERNED. ALTHOUGH NO-ONE LIKES BEING SICK, EACH ILLNESS HELPS BUILD KATE'S IMMUNE SYSTEM. SHE HAS NO QUALMS ABOUT KATE ATTENDING SCHOOL.

3.30 MANY CHILDREN OF THIS AGE HAVE NOT ACQUIRED IMMUNITY TO A NUMBER OF THE MOST COMMON DISEASES YET, AND KATE IS NO EXCEPTION. BY THE END OF THE DAY SHE HAS A SORE THROAT AND HER NOSE IS BECOMING BLOCKED.

12.45 AIRBORNE VIRUSES ARE HARD TO AVOID WHEN CHILDREN SNEEZE AND COUGH. DISEASE CAN ALSO BE PASSED ON BY CONTACT CONTAMINATION, AS WHEN KATE SHARES A DRINK WITH A COLD-RIDDEN FRIEND.

NEXT DAY BY KEEPING KATE AT HOME HER MOTHER CAN MAKE SURE KATE GETS REST AND PLENTY OF FLUIDS, AND SEES THE DOCTOR IF HER CONDITION GETS WORSE. SHE KNOWS THAT KATE IS INFECTIOUS AND DECIDES TO KEEP HER AWAY FROM HER BROTHERS WHO MIGHT CATCH THE BUG.

APPLE

Self-help for ENT problems

Illnesses of the ENT are some of the most common, and treatment is widely and readily available. Understanding the advantages and disadvantages of different treatments helps you to choose the most appropriate remedy.

OVER-THE-COUNTER DRUGS

Many medications intended for use in ear, nose and throat illness are available over the counter (OTC), without a doctor's prescription. However, some do need a trained pharmacist to be present in order for you to be able to buy them. Keep in mind that even drugs available over the counter can have side effects or may not be suitable for you. Always read the information on the pack or ask the pharmacist for advice.

Your medicine cabinet

A number of OTC drugs can effectively combat common symptoms. However, those for illness of the ears, nose and throat often contain more than you bargained for and you should be aware of pitfalls with these generally useful drugs.

Painkillers

Effective painkillers for treating headaches, sore throats, fever and general cold and flu symptoms include paracetamol, ibuprofen and aspirin. However, all can be dangerous if taken inappropriately.

Aspirin should not be given to children under 12 years old or taken if you are breastfeeding. It can cause gastric irritation and even ulceration. Those allergic to aspirin may develop life-threatening anaphylaxis and should carefully check the labels of cold remedies to avoid aspirin.

Paracetamol is extremely dangerous if the maximum safe and recommended dosage is exceeded – as few as 20 tablets taken in a 24-hour period can cause severe liver damage in an adult and, less frequently, acute kidney failure. If you suspect paracetamol overdose seek urgent medical help.

Ibuprofen can cause gastric irritation and, in theory, can worsen asthma. Those allergic to aspirin should not take ibuprofen or similar drugs, and neither should these drugs be taken during pregnancy or while breastfeeding. If you suffer from high blood pressure consult your doctor before starting the drug.

Cough remedies

A wide variety of cough remedies is available OTC, mainly containing various drugs in a flavoured syrup base. The effectiveness of cough remedies is doubtful, which is why they are rarely prescribed by doctors, and there is no hard evidence that expectorants – medicines that encourage sputum production in order to make it easier to cough up – are effective at all. Suppressants, which suppress the cough reflex, may be helpful at night because they contain codeine and similar drugs that may help get a good night's rest. However, these drugs can cause constipation. Also, codeine can be habit-forming and for this reason many pharmacists prefer it to be prescribed by a doctor.

positive health tips

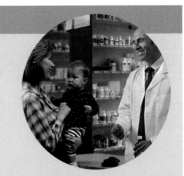

Using OTC medicines wisely

Before you take any medication, whether prescribed or purchased, you should always check the following:

- What is the correct dosage?

- Is the drug still in date? Many drugs have an expiry date printed somewhere in the packaging after which they may lose their efficacy or, in some cases, be dangerous to take.

- Are there instructions about when to take the drug (such as before or after food, or at bedtime)?

- Make sure you do not take different drugs with the same ingredients that could result in accidental overdose, or that do not interact well together. If in doubt, consult the pharmacist.

- How long is it safe to take a drug before seeking advice from a health professional? This should be printed on the packet.

- Keep medicines in a lockable cupboard out of reach of children, and check the contents regularly to dispose of out-of-date drugs.

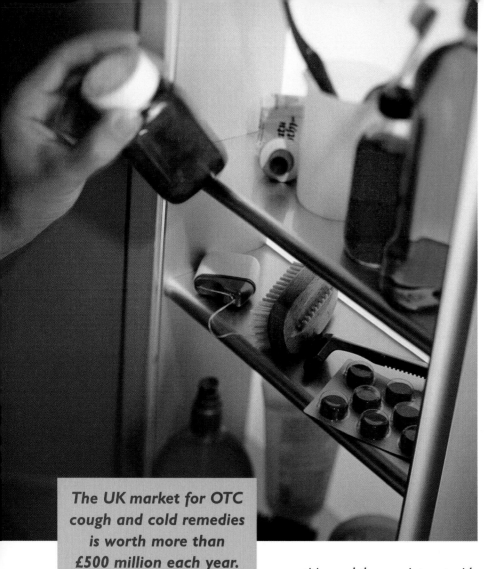

The UK market for OTC cough and cold remedies is worth more than £500 million each year.

Antihistamines
These are often contained in cold and flu remedies because they dry up mucus production. They are also useful in treating allergic conditions such as hay fever. Side effects include drowsiness, but this varies depending on which preparation you take.

Decongestants
These help to alleviate a blocked or runny nose and are available in tablet and capsule form, and as sprays, sticks and drops. They cease to be effective after a week, however, after which they can cause worsening of the original symptoms. Topical decongestant drugs can affect your heart rate and raise your blood pressure if absorbed in great enough quantities, and they can interact with other drugs. Therefore it is wise to avoid using them if possible.

Cold and flu remedies
There are many preparations available OTC, so it is worth talking to a pharmacist about their potential benefits and disadvantages. Some contain unhelpful ingredients, such as caffeine; others can be dangerous if they interact with other drugs. Some people have become addicted to these compound remedies. Dosage regimes can be complicated, overdoses dangerous, and generally it's easier to stick to individual drugs.

Eardrops
Various drops are available OTC. Some of these can make the skin sore after a few days' use and others are available to soothe irritated skin, but are not effective for earache. They never cure earache – you need to see a doctor to determine its cause.

Sore throat remedies
These are available as lozenges to suck and sprays for the throat. Most preparations available for a sore throat contain mixtures of antiseptic, flavourings and painkillers. Some sprays contain local anaesthetics, which not only deaden pain sensation but also perception of hot and cold – be careful not to burn your throat after using a spray.

MEDICINE FOR CHILDREN
Children can be far more sensitive to drugs than adults, so it is vital when administering drugs to children to read the labels carefully to find out dosage, delivery and timing, and follow the directions exactly. If at all unsure of any of the directions, contact your pharmacist. Only mix medications on your doctor's advice.

Use your pharmacist wisely

Cut down on unnecessary visits to the doctor by consulting a pharmacist first. A pharmacist will be able to give advice on:

- *Whether your symptoms are the result of a potentially serious condition or not.*

- *Whether another medication you are taking rules out a particular OTC remedy.*

- *If a remedy is suitable if you are pregnant or breastfeeding.*

COMPLEMENTARY THERAPIES

Recent years have seen a boom in the demand for complementary medicine as an increasing number of people develop resistance to antibiotics and turn to alternative methods for solutions to their medical problems.

Many schools of alternative medicine have roots in ancient tradition, and at the heart of all of them is an emphasis on the health and well-being of the whole body as the basis for curing or alleviating specific ailments. Fundamental is an awareness of what constitutes a healthy diet, and how what you eat may determine the optimal functioning of your immune system, which is vital in maintaining the good health of your ears, nose and throat (see page 64). In some cases, this may result in the elimination of entire food groups from the diet in order to alleviate or cure symptoms; this is a relatively new concept in conventional medicine.

Homeopathy

First developed in the late 18th century, homeopathy aims to enhance the body's natural tendency to heal itself. Patients are treated with minute doses of a plant, animal or mineral substance which would cause the same symptoms in a well person if taken in excess. In other words, homeopathy is the practice of treating like with like. Usually administered in pill form, treatments are so diluted as to be harmless to babies, children and during pregnancy. Homeopathy is a precise science with many remedies to treat most conditions, depending on what the specific symptoms are.

Aromatherapy

Treatment using scents can be traced back to the worlds of ancient Egypt and Greece. It involves the use of oils extracted from plants, flowers, seeds, barks, roots and leaves to provide physical and psychological therapeutic relief for a wide range of ailments.

All essential oils have natural healing properties which, once absorbed into the body either by inhalation or through the skin, display antiseptic qualities. Some act as anti-depressants, some as pain relievers, while others are anti-viral or anti-inflammatory. The attraction of such treatment is that the oils

Don't go it alone

Complementary therapies are not intended as a replacement for orthodox treatments, but should rather work with them in order to provide relief – hence the term complementary. You should always consult your GP before taking any course of action and should not rely on self-diagnosis. Complementary treatment is almost always tailored to suit an individual's needs, with the result that remedies for similar ailments may vary from person to person.

have a positive effect on the whole body – both mentally and physically – and without side effects if used properly. Different oils can be effective for different problems of the ears, nose and throat (see page 58). Add two to three drops of the appropriate oil to a tissue, place near your nose (not touching) and inhale. Or prepare a steam inhalation by adding five to seven drops of an oil to a bowl of just-boiled water. Hold

Homeopathic remedies for ear problems

SYMPTOMS	TREATMENT
Pain in the ears when babies are teething	Chamomilla 30 Every 2 hours for one day
Acute pain with discharge from the nose and ears	Mercuris solubillis 30 Every 2 hours for 2–3 days
Pain in the ears without deafness or discharge	Mullein oil 3–4 drops in the ear 2–3 times a day for one day
Pain with discharge from the ears	Pulsatilla 30 (right) Every 4 hours for 2 days

your face over the bowl and breathe deeply and rhythmically for several minutes. To intensify the effect, shroud your head and the bowl with a towel to trap the steam.

Western herbalism

Like aromatherapy, herbalism exploits the natural healing properties of plants, but herbal remedies are taken in a variety of forms, including tinctures, tablets, teas, compresses and also in their natural state. They can be used to alleviate many symptoms, or to prevent illness developing in the first place. Chewing on root ginger, for example, can alleviate or prevent travel sickness (see page 60).

Auricular therapy

While the most common complementary therapies concentrate on alleviating and curing coughs, colds and fevers, there is one school that focuses on the ears – auricular therapy. A branch of acupuncture, it works on the theory that there are some 300 points on energy channels on the ear, each of which represents a different part of the human body

and that any given pain can be alleviated by applying pressure – using either fingers or an acupuncture needle, or sometimes a laser or magnet – to the corresponding point on the ear. While auricular therapy deals for the most part with the body as a whole, some success has been reported in the relief and treatment of sinus problems and tinnitus.

Ten essential oils for ears, nose and throat

All of these oils except garlic may be added to a steam inhalation, which provides instant and lasting relief. Several may be gargled*. Garlic oil is applied as eardrops.

SYMPTOM OR CONDITION	ESSENTIAL OIL
Sinusitis, fever, nausea, vertigo	Peppermint
Common cold, flu	Lemon
Catarrh, common cold, cough, fever, flu, sinusitis	Eucalyptus
Common cold, flu, sinusitis, whooping cough	Tea tree
Common cold, flu, laryngitis, sore throat	Thyme*
Earache, whooping cough, vertigo	Lavender*
Cough, sore throat	Hyssop*
Earache	Garlic
Throat infections, sore throat, laryngitis, tonsillitis	Clary sage*
Earache, nausea	Chamomile

The auricular map
Auricular therapists believe that the ear is a map of an inverted body. Points representing the head and neck are generally located on or near the lobe, while those representing the feet are at the top of the external ear.

Different types of acupuncture
Auricular acupuncture differs from regular acupuncture because it works on pressure points to tap directly into the central nervous system, rather than opening the energy channels to release the flow of 'chi' or energy throughout the body.

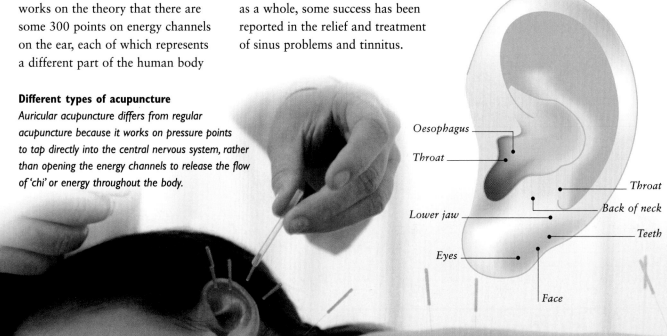

Oesophagus
Throat
Throat
Back of neck
Lower jaw
Teeth
Eyes
Face

Trouble-free travelling

Motion sickness is common but by no means inevitable. There are several tried-and-tested drugs as well as many common-sense precautions you can take to reduce your risk of suffering.

Also known as travel sickness or *mal de mer*, motion sickness is a common problem in childhood, that tends to be less of a nuisance as you get older. However, in severe sea swells, whole shiploads of people can be affected.

Research suggests that some people are seasick because they expect to be: conquering this feeling can keep you well.

WHAT CAUSES MOTION SICKNESS?

The symptoms are brought on when the brain receives conflicting messages from the sensory input of the eyes, the balance organs and the body's spatial receptors. For example, if you are travelling by car and reading at the same time, your eyes send the message to your brain that you are stationary, while your inner ear tells the brain that you are moving. This sets off a chain of self-perpetuating reactions in the unconscious part of the brain.

WHAT ARE THE SYMPTOMS?

The symptoms at their mildest include a feeling of discomfort and uneasiness. As things get worse you can start to feel sick and then develop headache, dizziness and tiredness. If the motion continues you can feel worse still, with sweating, pallor, yawning and hyperventilation all occurring. Vomiting is common and can be prolonged and severe.

Recent research has reported that a large number of US space shuttle astronauts suffer from motion sickness, particularly in the first two or three days of their mission. This is largely because of the repeated sudden head movements. Emotional factors and anxiety are also likely to be involved.

Research has been carried out on the effects of ginger root in combating 'space sickness', but biofeedback techniques seem to have the greatest effect on reducing motion sickness in space. Through these techniques, astronauts are taught to take control of bodily functions that are generally considered to be involuntary, such as monitoring breathing and heart rate.

BEATING TRAVEL SICKNESS

Being tired makes your body less able to cope with motion sickness, so try to get a good night's sleep before you travel.

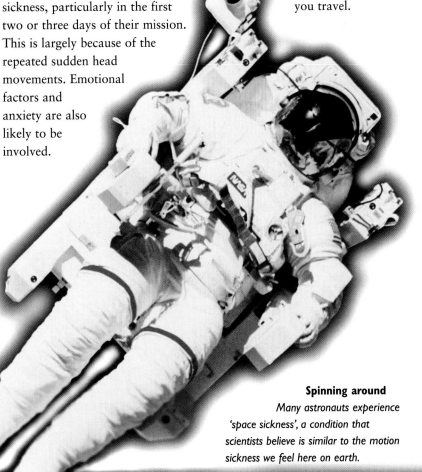

Spinning around
Many astronauts experience 'space sickness', a condition that scientists believe is similar to the motion sickness we feel here on earth.

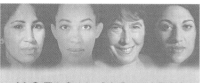

MOTION SICKNESS

Women are four times as likely as men to be seasick. Researchers have measured the stomach activity of men and women subjected to similar movements to those that induce motion sickness and, although they found comparable activity, the women were far more likely to say they felt sick. Research on round-the-world yachtswomen has shown that nausea is closely linked to the menstrual cycle, usually being worse in the three days before and first few days of a menstrual period, prompting theories that it may be linked to hormone levels.

Ginger: the travel drug?

There is some evidence that ginger – as tea, ale or as crystallised candy – has a beneficial effect on motion sickness. It is believed to act on the gastrointestinal system rather than on the balance mechanism.

Drugs

Drugs for travel sickness must be taken in advance.

You can buy some direct, while others are only available with a doctor's prescription. Some may cause drowsiness and you should note the risk of driving after taking these drugs. Some also interact with alcohol and other drugs affecting the brain. Hyoscine (marketed as Kwells and Junior Kwells) is the most effective, and is available over the counter in tablet form as well as in soluble tablets for children. It should not be taken if you have glaucoma, and it can cause drowsiness, visual disturbance and a dry mouth, although this is not usually a problem at the small doses involved. It is also available – by prescription only – as a patch that you stick onto your skin 5–6 hours before your journey (this is sold under the name Scopoderm). The effect lasts up to 72 hours, which is particularly useful on board ship. Antihistamine drugs also have an effect on motion sickness and are available for adults and children (they include Stugeron, Sea-legs and Avomine).

Pressure wrist bands

If you are wary of potential side effects of drugs, you could try elastic acupressure wrist bands. One is worn on each wrist, like a watch or sweatband, and incorporates a button attached to the inner side. This applies constant pressure to the P6 meridian point on each wrist and can considerably lessen the experience of motion sickness. Compared to most drugs, there are no side effects and the benefits are immediate – you simply put them on 5–10 minutes before you set off.

Break your journey

If it is possible, having a break in your journey can help your system to adjust and lessen feelings of motion sickness. This may add an hour to your journey but will be worth the delay.

Have a meal or snack

In some cases the fear of travel sickness puts a person off eating before travelling, which makes the situation worse. A light meal helps to settle the stomach before a journey and reduces the likelihood of motion sickness. Try to eat a small meal before setting out, but avoid spicy or fatty foods. Eating plain biscuits or crackers or sucking mints during the journey can also help.

Stay hydrated

Take frequent sips of water during the journey and, if you are sick, be sure to replace the fluids you have lost. Avoid alcohol and caffeine.

CHOOSE YOUR SEAT WISELY

Choosing where you sit can help to prevent or alleviate motion sickness. Always travel where your eyes will see the same motion that your inner ears and body will experience, to prevent conflicting messages being sent to the brain. So, for example, in a car, sit in the front and look forward. Do not attempt to read: even map reading can provoke feelings of sickness.

If possible, consider your environment before you travel: if you are going on a cruise and are prone to seasickness, choose your season of travel and geographical location with care. Try to avoid destinations where there is likely to be rough going, and make sure you will have the opportunity to sit out on deck.

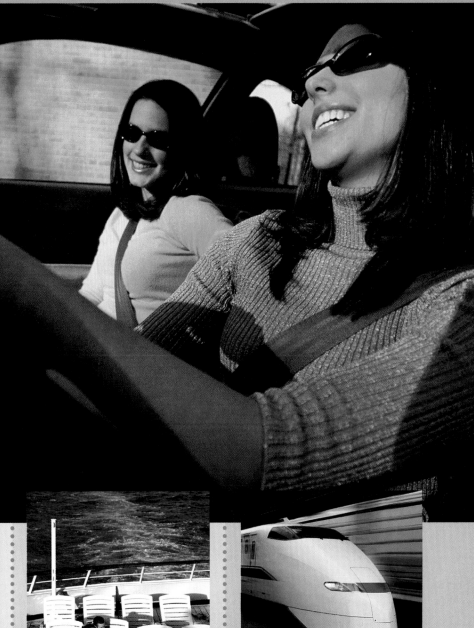

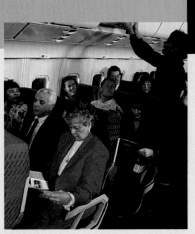

Flying high
If you tend to feel nauseous, try to choose a seat over the wing and sit by a window so that you can see the direction of travel. If the wing seats are gone, sit as near the middle of the plane as you can.

On board ship
To avoid sea sickness don't lie in your cabin, go on deck so that you can see the horizon. Bigger is definitely better when it comes to ships, and those with stabilisers are better still.

Rail travel
Those sensitive to motion sickness may find rail travel a problem, particularly on fast trains. If this applies to you, reserve a window seat facing the direction of travel and look out of the window.

EARS AND AIR PRESSURE

Ear problems related to a change in environmental air pressure are very common and can result in temporary pain and hearing loss.

When ears pop

The middle ear normally contains air at atmospheric pressure. Usually, when you swallow, air enters your middle ear from your mouth via the eustachian tube and is absorbed by the membrane lining the middle ear. In this way the pressure stays constant. If the eustachian tube is blocked for any reason, the middle ear pressure drops, pulling the eardrum inwards, stretching it and causing pain. If it remains blocked the middle ear starts to fill with fluid produced from the membrane lining the middle ear.

Air travel

When you travel by air your middle ear is exposed to rapid changes in air pressure and so you must swallow frequently to equalise the middle ear pressure – it pays to stay awake during take-off and landing in order to ensure this happens. Equalising the pressure cannot happen properly if your eustachian tubes are blocked, however, and if this happens you can experience discomfort.

Be alert

Maintaining constant pressure is also important in other situations when you change altitude rapidly such as during a deep-sea dive. Pilots and divers are taught to equalise pressure by practising regular controlled swallowing and other tricks devised to ensure that the eustachian tubes are kept open.

The Valsalva manoeuvre

If the natural methods on the right do not work, you can try the Valsalva manoeuvre: you may be accustomed to doing this without realising that the technique had an official name.

1 Hold your nostrils closed
2 Breathe in and close your mouth
3 Force air backwards into the back of your nose using your cheek and throat muscles.

If this is successful you will hear a pop and feel the pressure change in your middle ear. The manoeuvre can be repeated as often as necessary.

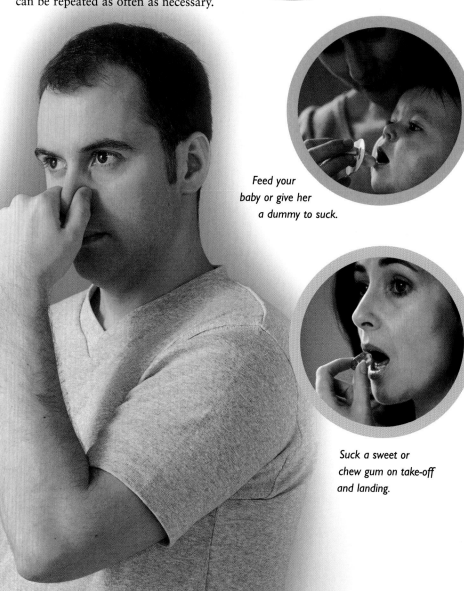

Natural ear 'poppers'
The different techniques used to equalise middle ear pressure vary only slightly, as they all use the same method of opening the eustachian tube.

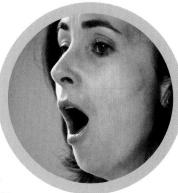

Yawn, or simply open your mouth wide, as if to yawn.

Feed your baby or give her a dummy to suck.

Suck a sweet or chew gum on take-off and landing.

HEALTHY LIVING FOR YOUR ENT

Lifestyle factors exert a great influence over the health of the whole body, including the ears, nose and throat. Every day we make choices that influence their health, including whether to smoke, what we eat, how much and what type of exercise we take, and whether we overstress the voice.

 64   *The ears, nose and throat are in constant contact with the outside world, so eating well to boost your immune system pays dividends.*

 66   *Antioxidants keep the body healthy – learn how easy it is to incorporate them into a varied diet.*

 68   *Your voice is your major means of communication with the outside world, so avoiding undue stress is vital.*

 72   *Discover the major negative impact that smoking, excessive drinking and illegal drugs can have on ENT health.*

 75   *A sense of balance is crucial to our sense of well-being. Learn how to maintain and improve this vital skill.*

 77   *Exercising in the heat or cold, and playing certain sports, affects your ears, nose and throat. Read how to protect yourself.*

Foods for healthy ENT

The health of the ears, nose and throat is dependent on a balanced diet with an emphasis on a few specific vitamins and nutrients that help to boost our ability to fight off infections and pollutants.

The close link between the ears, nose and throat means that, once one area suffers from an infection, the others may well follow. While there aren't any specific foods to boost the health of individual organs within the ENT system, a balanced diet plays an important role in maintaining their overall health – in particular, a diet that focuses on maintaining optimum health of the immune system.

KEEPING THE BALANCE

The simplest way to maintain a balanced diet is to remember the recommended ratios to one another of the five different groups that make up the foods we eat. The first group includes bread, cereals and potatoes, providers of carbohydrates and fibre, and should form the basis of your diet, with 6 to 11 portions a day. Fruit and vegetables, excellent sources of vitamin C, carotenes, folates and fibre, make up the next group, from which you should aim to eat five servings a day. Balance this with two portions of milk and dairy foods – for calcium, protein, vitamins B_{12}, A and D – and two portions of meat or fish (or four of pulses or tofu), for protein, iron, the B vitamins, zinc and magnesium. Finally, include only a sparing number of foods that contain fat and sugar. Once this basic diet is established, you will be able to concentrate on the foods that contribute specifically to the health of your ears, nose and throat.

MAINTAINING A HEALTHY MUCOUS MEMBRANE

Any airborne irritant that escapes the automatic filtering of the nose encounters the mucous membrane that lines the passages of the nose and throat. Keeping this membrane healthy is vital for fighting infections.

Vitamin B_2

Vitamin B_2 or riboflavin contributes to the health of the mucous membrane, and rich sources include liver, milk, cheese, yogurt, eggs, green vegetables, yeast extract and fortified breakfast cereals. A viscous substance produced by the mucous membrane traps foreign bacteria and destroys it using a chemical called lysozyme. A deficiency of vitamin B_2 causes a change to the mucous membrane and this process may slow down, so weakening the strength of the nose's defence against bacteria, and exposing the body to a greater risk of infection to the epiglottis, tonsils, pharynx or larynx.

Vitamin A

An important vitamin for optimum functioning of the mucous membrane, vitamin A can be found in two forms: as retinol in foods from animals, and as carotenoids in foods from plant sources. Animal sources of vitamin A include milk, fortified margarine, butter, cheese, egg yolk, liver and fatty fish such as salmon, mackerel, kippers and trout. Vegetable sources of vitamin A include carrots, tomatoes and dark green vegetables.

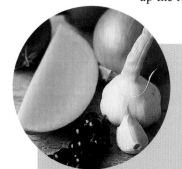

ENT *SUPERFOODS*

All whole, unprocessed foods are good for the immune system, helping it to fight off infections, but some foods are particularly effective at keeping your ears, nose and throat in good health.

MUESLI Packed with B vitamins – including the all-important B_{12} – muesli and other whole-grain cereals mixed with nuts, seeds and dried fruits, is a good provider of minerals and vitamins.
SALMON Like many oily fish, salmon is a reliable source of the antioxidants vitamin E and selenium.
BLACKCURRANTS Amazingly, these tiny currants are one of the richest sources of vitamin C, with 100g (4oz) of fruit yielding approximately 200mg.
MANGO This is the best fruit source of antioxidant carotenoids, and one of the very few fruit sources of vitamin E.
ONION Along with **GARLIC,** onion contains natural antibiotics which are believed to bring relief from the symptoms of colds and flu.

HEALTHFUL ANTIOXIDANTS

Although colds and flu are spread rapidly from one person to the next, you are more likely to succumb if your immune system is weak. This leaves you with lower resistance for fighting infections. They key to optimum functioning of the immune system is a good intake of antioxidants, essential for 'mopping up' free radicals. Antioxidants include vitamins C and E, carotenoids (plant sources of vitamin A) and the minerals selenium, zinc and magnesium, which protect the body's cells from being damaged by free radicals. Zinc plays a particularly important role in the functioning of the immune system, and a deficiency is associated with a range of immunological defects, although they can be reversed once there is adequate zinc in the diet.

What are free radicals?

Free radicals are produced by the body's normal metabolic processes and, if they are allowed to build up, they can cause damage to key components in the body such as DNA (the cell's building blocks), protein and fat. Cells in which damage to the DNA is not repaired are more likely to develop cancer. Free radicals can also oxidise polyunsaturated fatty acids in foods and in cell membranes in the body to compounds called peroxides which can damage cells. Antioxidants inhibit the oxidation of polyunsaturated fatty acids.

HELPING A COLD

Certain foods and drinks may help to alleviate cold symptoms in the ears, nose and throat and can offer a natural alternative to OTC drugs.

Honey and lemon drink

It is likely that any warm drink will have a soothing effect on inflamed surfaces, and thus provide relief from a sore throat and cough. A sweet and bitter hot drink, most commonly containing honey and lemon, is likely to be more tasty during a time when the sense of taste is affected. Honey has antiseptic and expectorant qualities that may also contribute to alleviating a sore throat, while lemon is rich in vitamin C.

Menthol

Menthol is a component of cornmint, peppermint and eucalyptus oils and has been used over the centuries to provide relief from nasal congestion. Nowadays, menthol is commonly contained in cough lozenges and helps to relieve the discomfort a cold can cause by imparting a cooling sensation that is felt in the nose and throat. The effect is temporary, rather like that of a localised anaesthetic.

Garlic

Garlic contains a compound called ajoene, which may have antibacterial effects, and allicin, a powerful natural antibiotic. Both of these substances are thought to prevent the common cold and relieve troublesome symptoms.

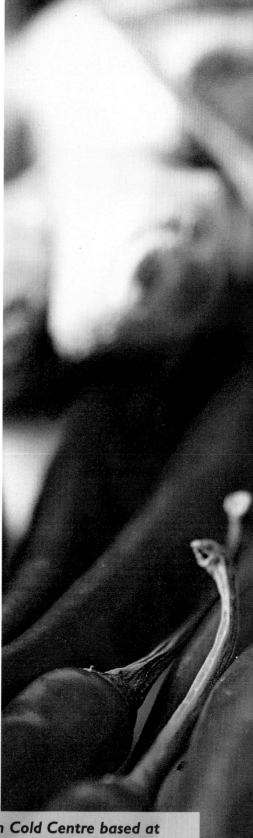

According to the Common Cold Centre based at Cardiff University, spicy and hot foods, particularly those including ginger and chilli, are decongestants, promoting airway secretions which can have a calming effect on an inflamed throat.

A good week for antioxidants

It is not difficult to enjoy a delicious diet rich in antioxidants – they are readily available in many of the foods found in our supermarkets and shops. The key is knowing which foods, and how best to combine them to achieve a healthy and balanced diet. This week of menus should start you off with some ideas.

Some easy ways to increase the antioxidants in your diet include:

- Start the day with a bowl of wholegrain cereal and semi-skimmed milk
- Snack on nuts, dried fruits, crispbread or flapjack
- Eat vegetable soup for lunch
- Replace a cup of tea or coffee with a citrus fruit juice
- Add a fresh salad to your evening meal

positive health tips

The best sources of antioxidants

- Vitamin C: fresh fruit – especially citrus fruits and blackcurrants, green vegetables and potatoes.
- Vitamin E: vegetable oils, nuts, vegetables and cereals.
- Carotenoids: carrots, tomatoes and dark green vegetables.
- Selenium: wholegrain cereals, meat, fish, offal, cheese and eggs.
- Zinc: milk, cheese, meat, eggs, fish, wholegrain cereals and pulses.
- Magnesium: wholegrain cereals, nuts and spinach.

Day One
BREAKFAST

Glass of orange juice
2 slices of wholemeal toast with blackcurrant jam
Herbal tea
LUNCH
Carrot and coriander soup
Slice of wholemeal bread
Natural yoghurt
SUPPER
Grilled chicken breast with brown rice
Tomato, mango, pepper and onion salsa

Day Two
BREAKFAST

Glass of grapefruit juice
Muesli with extra sunflower seeds and semi-skimmed milk
Lemon tea
LUNCH
Egg mayonnaise, spinach and tomato sandwich with wholemeal bread
Orange
SUPPER
Poached salmon, brown rice and broccoli
Green salad with nuts

Day Three
BREAKFAST
2 soft-boiled eggs
2 slices of granary bread
Lemon tea
LUNCH
Tuna and sweetcorn sandwich with wholemeal bread
Apple
SUPPER
Pork fillet kebab
Spinach, onion and chickpea salad
Fruit salad

Day Four
BREAKFAST

Glass of orange juice
Bowl of All Bran with handful of berries
LUNCH
Crab and avocado salad
French bread
SUPPER
Lentils with rice and celery
Green salad

Day Five
BREAKFAST

Half a grapefruit
Muesli with semi-skimmed milk
Herbal tea
LUNCH
Cream cheese and tomato sandwich with wholemeal bread
Orange, peach or nectarine
SUPPER
Mussels with white wine, garlic and herbs
French bread
Green salad

Day Six
BREAKFAST
Melon and papaya fruit salad
2 slices of granary toast with marmalade
Herbal tea
LUNCH
Mixed bean salad
French bread
SUPPER
Lamb chops
Roasted aubergine and red pepper
Tomato and onion salad

Day Seven

BREAKFAST

*Greek yoghurt with
mixed berries*

*2 slices of wholemeal toast
with honey*

LUNCH

Root vegetable soup

2 slices of rye bread

SUPPER

*Grilled tuna with pesto-mashed
potato*

Rocket, tomato and cucumber salad

*Natural yoghurt with honey and
hazelnuts*

HEALTHY SNACKS

Antioxidant-rich snacks can help to boost your intake. Keep some of the following handy for mid morning or afternoon snacks.

Piece of fresh fruit	Fresh vegetables
Small bowl of fruit salad	Boiled egg
Handful of dried fruit	Small tub of yoghurt
Handful of nuts	Portion of frozen yoghurt or ice cream
Handful of seeds	Piece of cheese
Wholemeal bread	Cup of tea
Crispbread	Glass of freshly squeezed fruit juice
Small bowl of cereal	Glass of milk

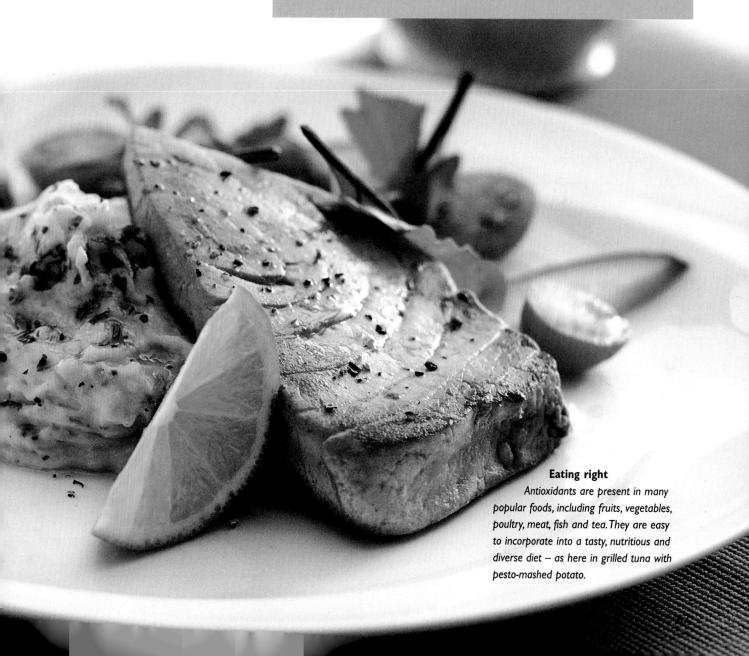

Eating right

Antioxidants are present in many popular foods, including fruits, vegetables, poultry, meat, fish and tea. They are easy to incorporate into a tasty, nutritious and diverse diet – as here in grilled tuna with pesto-mashed potato.

Taking care of your voice

Stressing your voice on a regular basis can damage the vocal cords, leading to permanent hoarseness. Furthermore, when the rest of your body is stressed your voice can suffer. Learning to relax your voice is the key to keeping it healthy.

Stress can be thought of in two ways. Firstly, the emotional response to a situation can manifest itself in stress if there is a feeling of lack of control. This is the 'fight or flight' response which prepares your body for action: whichever you choose your voice may come into play. Shouting may increase the aggression which is helping you to fight, or draw attention to others that you are going to flee. Secondly, you can consciously choose to place your body under stress in order to maximise its response, for example when running a race or when singing an opera.

These are both examples of physiological stress, a condition that occurs when the body is asked to perform activities far outside its regular functioning capacity. This is a situation that is often demanded of the voice – just think of the number of times in the past week that you have raised your voice in speech, or in song, louder than necessary – and it is harmful to the vocal cords.

INSTANT DAMAGE

Your vocal cords are highly sensitive in order to produce the range of sounds they do, and extreme stress can have an instant, and sometimes prolonged, effect on them.

Shouting down the house

When you shout with too much force, it is possible to damage the lining of your vocal cords, causing hoarseness. The muscles to your throat tighten and breathing becomes shallower as a reaction to the excessive tension. This results in more effort being exerted to recover your voice, which can make it worse. If the voice isn't given time to recover from stress – if you shout while your voice is still hoarse and your throat is still sore – you risk

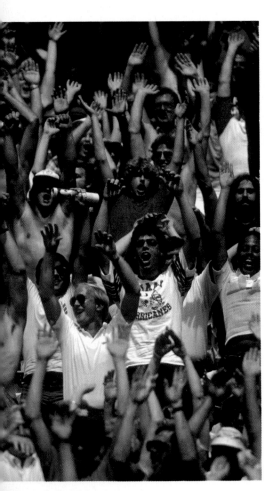

Roaring crowds
Persistent shouting can lead to the development of vocal cord nodules, and a permanently hoarse or breathy voice.

damaging the vocal cords still further. If you find yourself regularly shouting in anger or frustration, getting help to sort out what is stressing you makes more sense than risking your voice. People who regularly stress their voices may need speech therapy to train them out of poor voice habits.

Clearing your throat

A lot of people cough and clear their throats when they are stressed. If this is done too aggressively, it can also result in vocal cord damage. It is much better to try to relax your throat by swallowing instead, as well as having sips of water.

Reflux

Stress can also result in acid reflux, where stomach acid flows up towards the larynx, causing discomfort and sometimes a voice disorder. To reduce reflux, give your body enough time to digest your food properly before rushing around, try not to eat hurriedly, and don't eat immediately before going to bed.

Sounding stressed

A stressed voice may sound more aggressive, inviting negative reactions from others, and breathing may become shallower as the pace of speaking gets quicker. If you can take the tension out of your voice you're more likely to breathe better and produce more efficient speech, and get a better response.

LONG-TERM DAMAGE

Sometimes damage is the result of soldiering on without observing signals telling you to relax. These include hoarseness and sore throat, as well as tension in your body.

EXERCISES TO RELAX A TENSE VOICE

1 *Before working directly on your voice, focus on your whole body. Look for tension in your knees, back, abdomen and face, all of which can accumulate to inhibit your natural ability to produce a healthy voice.*

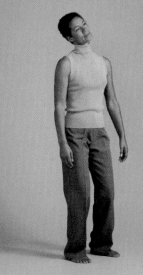

2 *Now try this exercise from the Alexander technique. Lie on your back on the floor, support your head with a cushion or pillow, and bring your knees up, keeping your feet on the floor. Allow yourself to feel heavy, close your eyes and focus on slow, gentle breathing. Try tensing and then letting go of different groups of muscles around your body to increase your awareness of tension. Now gently roll your head from side to side to release tension in your neck; this should make your voice feel freer and easier to use.*

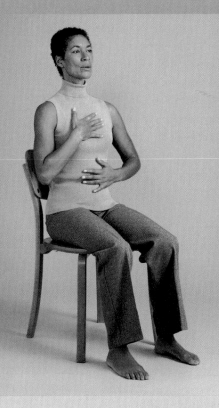

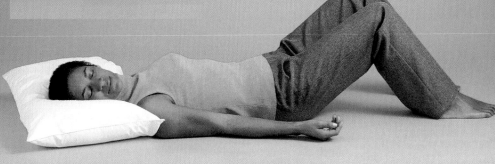

3 *Sit upright on a chair, and put one hand on your chest and one on your abdomen. Breathe in to the bottom of your lungs and feel both hands move out; if you find yourself gulping air, slow down your breathing. Inhale through your nose as slowly as you can, aiming to get to a count of ten, then exhale just as slowly. If you hear a harsh whisper when you breathe in, this is because you are narrowing your throat and tensing your vocal cords too much. This exercise should make you aware of the coordination between breathing and speaking.*

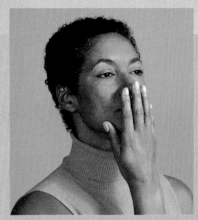

4 *Practise humming a single note. You should feel a buzzing sensation in your lips and eventually your face; if you can't feel it, try placing your fingers lightly over your face and nose. This encourages you to project your voice and create greater resonance by taking the effort away from your vocal cords.*

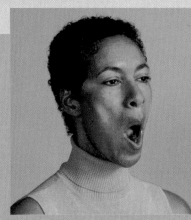

5 *Try humming a continuous note while clenching your teeth. Your voice will sound trapped, thin and nasal. Now start making a chewing motion, which relaxes the jaw, and notice how the sound becomes bigger and moves forward in your mouth.*

Be career wise

Certain jobs carry greater risks for the voice than others. The traditional regimental sergeant major fairly obviously stresses his voice on a daily basis, but singers, teachers, lawyers, clergymen, aerobics instructors and politicians regularly risk voice damage.

The problem is compounded in some cases by environmental factors: the atmosphere in many classrooms, for example, is dry, which is unkind to the throat. In addition, many public buildings are built without the advice of an acoustician, so professionals may have to fill a space that was not designed for a single human voice. Noise, too, makes matters worse. Studies have shown that we tend to raise our voices by about 3dB for every 10dB increase in ambient noise level. Since the noise level in an average nursery class can be as high as 80dB, it is hardly surprising that teachers suffer from voice problems.

If you belong to one of these at-risk groups, it's important to be especially kind to your larynx.

An American survey found that although teachers make up only 4 per cent of the US work force, they form 20 per cent of patients at voice clinics.

Careful karaoke

Singers are prone to voice problems because of the extra effort they use in the throat when singing. Professional singers are taught to warm the voice before rehearsing or performing, singing mid-range notes before gradually working towards those at the top and bottom of their ranges, and practising scales and arpeggios, as well as breathing exercises to help in efficient, unstrained sound production.

Amateurs, however, may not take such care. Vocal difficulties often arise from a poorly produced loud voice, intended to fill a pub or hall. Such sounds can easily result in bruised vocal cords. It is wise not to sing without warming the voice as described above, especially if you have a sore throat, as you will be vulnerable to inflammation of the vocal cords.

Even with training, professionals face problems:

- Overuse of the vocal cords through extensive rehearsal and performance schedules.
- Travel, particularly by air which is noisy and tiring, as well as involving sitting in a pressurised, low-humidity environment, can stress even a professional's voice.
- As with sportspeople, singers need to acclimatise to high altitudes before they can perform without risking voice stress.
- The atmosphere in many auditoriums is cold, dry and dusty, which can harm the vocal cords.
- Some clubs and small venues allow smoking, which compromises performers' voices.

To club or not to club

If you are going out to a club or concert where the music is loud, accept that you are not going to be able to chat too. Average noise levels are too loud to shout over. The

---

positive health tips

Be kind to your larynx: how to look after your voice

- If your job involves talking a lot, make sure you have quiet periods in the day.

- Don't talk above loud background noise if you don't have to.

- If you find you are often shouting as a means of dealing with anger, consider counselling or assertiveness training.

- Don't overdo spicy foods. These can cause laryngeal irritation.

- Steer clear of chemicals that might irritate your throat, such as aerosol sprays and household cleaning products.

- Avoid smoking and excessive drinking.

- Don't sit hunched over your computer keyboard or desk. This puts a strain on your neck muscles, which are important in voice production.

- Don't spend too long in dry, cold air. The larynx likes to be wet and warm. Steam inhalation will thin out mucus trapped in the nose and throat.

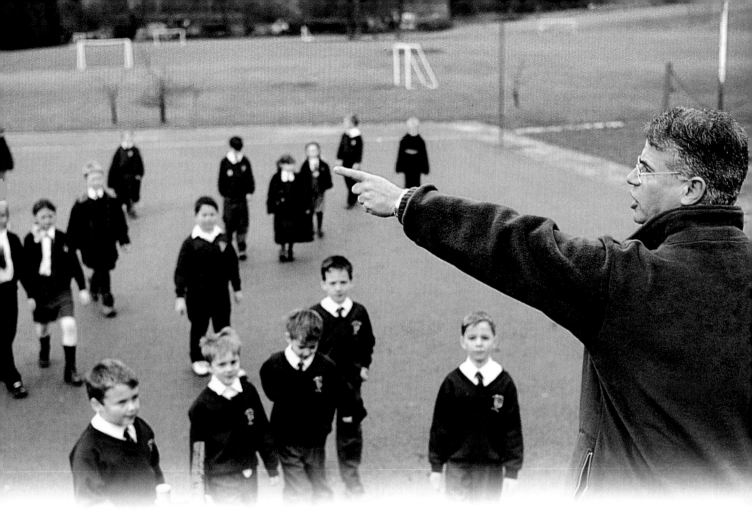

Controlling presence

Teachers who manage to maintain a disciplined atmosphere through their presence, rather than relying on shouting above the din of the playground, risk less voice stress than their colleagues.

atmosphere in such venues may be smoky, too, which will also affect your throat and voice.

Unclench that jaw

If you are overly tense you may grind your teeth at night, resulting in a clenched jaw. This is another very common cause of vocal tension, making the voice sound 'held back' or muffled. If you find yourself swallowing your sounds and having to make an extra effort with your throat to compensate for not being heard, you may need to take steps to undo the tension. We all clench our jaws and grit our teeth when we are feeling stressed – the expression 'I had to grit my teeth' comes from having to restrain tension and frustration – but it should not become almost permanent.

Be socially wise

Two of the most common social stress relievers, smoking and alcohol, both dry out the voice and irritate the larynx, resulting in deepening, hoarseness and other changes. Some people find this sexy – and some performers cultivate this style – but in the long run it ages the voice.

Keep lubricated

Stress can result in your neglecting to eat when you need to, or not drinking enough fluids throughout the day, which results in dehydration and a dry throat.

IT'S NOT TRUE!

'If the vocal cords are healthy, the voice is too'

Your voice does not depend solely on healthy vocal cords, but on a combination of three things working together:

- breathing, which provides the necessary power;
- the moving vocal cords, which are the source of the sound;
- your mouth and facial structures, which act as a filter, changing the size and shape of the sound.

If you spread your lips, your voice sounds brighter, whereas if you round them, it comes out deeper and duller.

Harmful habits

Some of the lifestyle habits that many people consider to be an integral part of a 'normal' social life can seriously damage your entire body, including your ears, nose and throat.

Social drugs fall into two broad categories: legal drugs such as tobacco and alcohol, and illegal, or street, drugs, including cannabis, cocaine and solvents.

TOBACCO SMOKING
Smoking tobacco causes a variety of disorders in the ears, nose and throat. These range from relatively minor problems, such as heavy snoring, to fatal cancers of the nose and throat. Choosing not to smoke can prevent, or at least significantly reduce, the risk of developing some of the following health problems.

Airway damage
The airways from the nose and mouth to the lungs are lined with a layer of mucus which helps to keep them clean and lubricated. This mucus contains antibodies to kill germs and is kept moving by a layer of tiny hair-like tissues called cilia. These hairs need a continuous supply of oxygen to function properly, but tobacco smoke restricts oxygen supply, paralysing the cilia so that they no longer perform the essential clearing action. Long-term smoking makes the paralysis permanent, so that mucus has to be coughed up: the result is the typical 'smoker's cough'.

Coughs and colds
People who smoke are more susceptible to coughs and colds because the immune system is harmed by tobacco smoke. For the same reason, they often suffer worse symptoms and take longer to get over colds than non-smokers.

Smoking is associated with an increased risk of acute and chronic rhinitis (inflammation of the mucus membrane lining the nose). Smokers are also at greater risk of sinusitis – inflammation of the tissues lining the sinus cavities – the condition often improves if people stop smoking.

Snoring
Heavy smokers are more likely to snore. Children exposed to environmental tobacco smoke (passive smoking) are also more likely to snore and the more smoke they are exposed to, the greater the likelihood they will snore. Experts have found that if one parent smokes, a child is roughly twice as

Understanding the risks
Schools and youth and community groups regularly invite police officers or counsellors from charitable organisations to discuss the legal, social and health implications of drink and drug use.

likely to snore than if their parent doesn't smoke, and if both parents smoke the child's risk of snoring nearly quadruples.

Mouth and throat cancer
There is a strong association between cancer of the mouth or throat and smoking. It is estimated that about 75 per cent of mouth and throat cancers are caused by tobacco use, and heavy use of both tobacco and alcohol increases risk dramatically. Tobacco smoke contains thousands of different chemicals which are

One study found that middle-aged men who smoked more than 15 cigarettes a day were six and a half times more likely than non-smokers to be frequent snorers.

released into the air as particles and gases. At least 40 of these are known to cause cancer, including benzene, formaldehyde and carbon monoxide. Although some chemicals are present in only tiny quantities, the cumulative effect of inhaling this cocktail of toxic compounds causes cancer.

While the lungs are the principal organs for the absorption of oxygen and other chemicals, some absorption also takes place in the nose and mouth. In fact, the nose is so efficient at absorbing substances into the bloodstream that some forms of medication are given in an aerosol formulation taken by nose.

Hearing loss

Smokers experience sudden hearing loss an average of 16 years earlier than people who have never smoked.

In addition, smokers are more likely than non-smokers to experience recurrent sudden hearing loss: 46 per cent of smokers suffer such a recurrence, while just 33 per cent of non-smokers do.

While experts are not sure how smoking increases a person's risk of hearing loss caused by exposure to loud noise, they believe decreased blood flow to the ears may play a role. The inner ear contains sensory cells and other tissues critical to hearing and the vessels that carry blood to the inner ear can become blocked by atherosclerosis (fatty plaques that adhere to the blood vessel walls). Furthermore, some researchers believe that high levels of carbon monoxide in the blood of smokers may directly damage sensory cells in the inner ear. Hearing loss is also directly related to ageing, and while this type of loss is common, there is some evidence that smoking may accelerate it.

ALCOHOL AND THE BODY

Alcohol affects all the body systems, especially the brain and liver. Over-indulgence carries significant health hazards, but there could be some significant health benefits associated with low or moderate consumption.

Ear, nose and throat damage

Alcohol consumption is associated with a number of cancers of the nose and throat, particularly in smokers. Alcohol is not a carcinogen in standard laboratory tests, but it may act as a 'co-carcinogen' or tumour

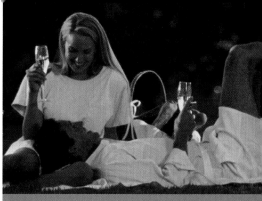

Drinking to your health

Moderate alcohol consumption on a regular basis is considered by many to be beneficial to overall health. Experts argue about the definition of moderate consumption, but generally agree that one or two standard drinks per day, depending on your gender and body weight, seem to lessen the chances of coronary heart disease and cardiovascular disease. Evidence also seems to show that moderate drinking can reduce the risk of kidney stones and osteoporosis, and help in the prevention of Alzheimer's disease.

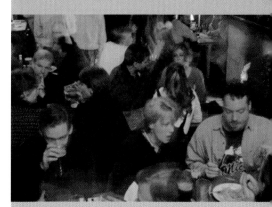

... or ill health?

Studies suggest that drinking alcohol increases the risk of cancers of the mouth, pharynx and larynx; the more consumed, the greater the risk. These risks are further multiplied by smoking: drinking four units of alcohol a day doubles the risk of oral and pharyngeal cancer, but combined with 20 cigarettes a day, the risk is quadrupled. A person who smokes 40 cigarettes a day has 15 times the cancer risk of a non-smoker and non-drinker.

promoter by irritating the lining of the gastrointestinal tract, making it more susceptible to the carcinogens in cigarette smoke.

ILLEGAL DRUGS

Illegal drug habits that are potentially damaging to the ears, nose or throat include smoking cannabis, snorting cocaine and inhaling solvents. Some of these drugs are harmful in the long term; others can do instant damage.

Cannabis

The harmful effects of smoking cannabis are similar to those of smoking tobacco, although people tend to smoke less cannabis than tobacco. Instant bodily reactions can be a dry mouth, throat, nose and eyes. Possible permanent damage takes the form of cancer. Cannabis contains more carcinogens than tobacco smoke,

and more tar. Furthermore, it is usually inhaled deeper into the lungs and held there for longer. For these reasons, some experts consider it even more likely to cause cancer than tobacco smoke.

Cocaine

Cocaine can cause both permanent and temporary damage to the body, depending on the method of use.

Snorting cocaine is particularly harmful to the nose and throat. The drug is absorbed into the bloodstream through the nasal tissues, causing a stuffy or runny nose, sinus problems, loss of smell, chapped nostrils, nose bleeds, sores around the nostrils, difficulty swallowing and hoarseness.

Prolonged snorting of cocaine can ulcerate the mucous membrane of the nose, and damage the nasal septum causing it to collapse. Since cocaine has anaesthetic qualities, users may not even realise the damage being done to their nose and mouth.

Nose and throat symptoms of smoking cocaine include dry lips and throat, hoarseness and a cough, which signals the damage being inflicted on the lungs.

Inhalants

An inhaled substance reaches the brain faster than anything that is injected, and the body's reaction to

Inadvertent damage
Many DIY products contain substances that produce a 'high'. If at all possible use these products outdoors and wear a facemask to protect your nose and throat. If you must work indoors, ensure good ventilation.

Passive smoking

Children who are exposed to tobacco smoke are particularly susceptible to ear infections, which may in turn lead to deafness. They also have more sore throats, blocked noses, hoarseness, and trouble getting over colds than other children, and are more likely to require surgery to remove the adenoids and tonsils. Children of smokers are 30 to 80 per cent more likely than children of non-smokers to have chronic cough or phlegm production. This is especially true for preschool children, who may spend more hours each day in a smoky environment.

inhalant fumes is potentially deadly. The immediate effects of inhalants on the nose and throat result from the body trying desperately to filter out the chemicals before they are allowed to reach the lungs and brain. Such effects can include sneezing, coughing, nosebleeds, decreased sense of smell and depressed breathing. Signs of solvent abuse include a red or running nose, sores around the mouth and nose and bad breath.

Hundreds of substances can be inhaled. They include adhesives, aerosols such as spray paint and hair spray, and anaesthetics such as nitrous oxide, or laughing gas, found in whipped cream canisters. Cleaning products such as dry cleaning fluid or spot remover, and solvents such as nail polish remover, paint thinner and remover and lighter fluid are also commonly abused substances.

Balancing acts

Good balance is essential in practically everything we do, from climbing stairs and lifting a child to riding a bike or carrying a cup of tea. Whatever age you are, it is always possible to improve your balance through regular exercise.

Like so many aspects of our health, we tend to take our sense of balance for granted, only really noticing it when we experience a problem. Both the ears and eyes play important roles in maintaining balance, sending different but complementary messages for the brain to interpret.

The balancing elite
Snowboarders require particularly good balance and coordination, attributes which combine to provide vital spatial awareness.

BALANCE AND SPORTS

If you exercise regularly you are undoubtedly working on your balance without necessarily realising it. Walking, using a treadmill and riding a road bike all require balance and coordination; more obviously, activities such as yoga or ice skating and skiing require good balancing skills. Sports scientists believe that the abilities to move and balance, as well as reaction times, are inextricably linked and all are crucial

to successful sports performance. If balance starts to become a problem, you should talk either to a fitness trainer at the local gym, or to a physiotherapist. Both these professionals can devise a series of exercises or suggest sporting activities to suit your balance problem, age and state of health. There is no need to give up exercise.

WHEN BALANCE IS A PROBLEM

Everyday causes of dizziness, such as a rapid head movement, motion sickness, and excess alcohol consumption, do not persist for long and are not necessarily of concern. There are more permanent causes of dizziness, however, that have lasting implications for well-being, and these include labyrinthitis, Menière's disease, vertigo and chronic middle ear infection. All these need professional medical advice and you should consult a doctor if you have prolonged dizziness with no obvious cause, or if dizziness interferes with your regular daily routine.

If you have vertigo

For sufferers of vertigo and other vestibular complaints, there are a series of exercises that specifically address the problem of balance. The Cawthorne-Cooksey exercises, derived from British surgeon Terence

Cawthorne's research into balance and movement therapy in the 1940s, form the basis of accepted treatment for sufferers of dizziness. These exercises need to be repeated twice daily on a regular basis, and initially should be carried out under the supervision of a physiotherapist.

positive health tips

Beating balance problems

- If you feel dizzy, hold on to something firm. Keep your eyes closed or focused on an immobile object and avoid moving your head.

- Your doctor may prescribe tablets or injections to reduce signals travelling from the ears to the brain during a dizzy spell.

- Cut down on alcohol, caffeine and salt: although this does not help all forms of dizziness, it does reduce the severity of symptoms in many cases.

- Avoid stress. Find ways to deal with stressful situations, such as stress management techniques, or try yoga or meditation.

- Don't make radical lifestyle changes. Dizzy spells may mean that you need to curtail certain activities, but don't stop doing things you enjoy.

- Get support. There are many support groups, both local and on the Internet, for sufferers from chronic dizziness. Their members know how you feel and will have positive advice and tips to help you to cope.

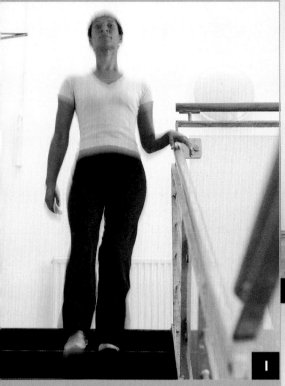

1

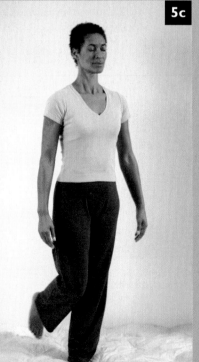

2

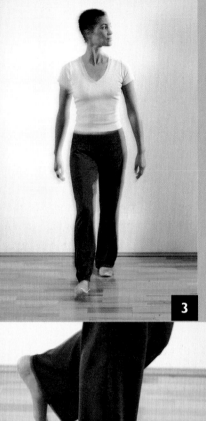

3

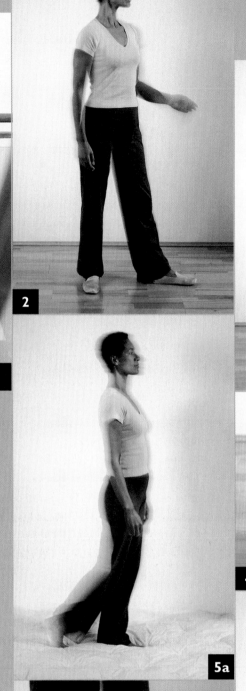

5a

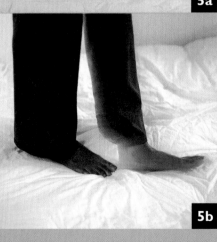

5b

5c

Balance for all

These Cawthorne-Cooksey exercises, in addition to helping those with balance problems, are useful for anyone who wants to improve balance in general.

1 Walk up and down stairs carefully with your eyes open, then repeat with your eyes closed. Hold onto a handrail for safety, if needed, especially with the eyes closed.

2 While standing, practise making sudden 90-degree turns, first with the eyes open, then closed.

3 While walking look side to side. A supermarket is a good place to do this – read labels as you walk down the aisle.

4 Practise standing on one foot. Do this with your eyes open, then closed. Repeat with the other foot.

5 Standing on a soft surface such as a mattress, pillow, or foam mat:
a. First walk across the surface to get used to it.
b. Walk heel to toe across the surface, first with the eyes open, then closed.
c. Practise standing on one foot with your eyes open, then closed.

Stay healthy while exercising

In moderation, all sports and activities are beneficial to your health and well-being, but there are some instances where there are extra benefits for the ears, nose and throat – and others where it is advisable to take special care.

Many sports and exercise activities improve or help you to maintain your balancing skills, but few specifically promote the health of your ears, nose and throat. Nonetheless, exercise is a great booster for the immune system, and will help to prevent the niggling and sometimes painful infections that affect these organs.

There are also some precautions and protective measures you should take when undertaking some sports.

COLD WEATHER PRECAUTIONS

Starting to exercise outdoors in cold weather can cause problems for your ears, nose and throat. An increased demand for oxygen can make you breathe more cold air in through

A chill in the air
Modern thermal headware uses lightweight materials that breathe, allowing you to cover your nose and throat when you need to.

your nose and mouth, triggering irritation. If the cold air hurts your throat, wrap a scarf over your nose and mouth until you are thoroughly warm. Protect your ears with a hat. If exercise-induced asthma is a problem, take every precaution and use your medication as your management plan indicates.

WARM WEATHER PRECAUTIONS

Hot, dry air not only dehydrates the body, it also dries out the mucous membrane of the nose, which may compromise the nose's ability to filter dust. Your throat too is likely to suffer in extremely dry weather. Sip water throughout any exercise session in hot, dry weather.

WATER SPORTS

Frequent swimming and water sports can be problematic for the ears, particularly in children. The most

common risk is swimmer's ear, an infection of the outer ear canal. Water enters the ear during swimming, carrying with it potentially damaging bacteria or fungus particles. The water usually runs out again and the ear dries leaving no risk from micro-organisms. When the water stays in the ear, however, the ear does not dry out properly, providing a perfect wet and warm breeding ground for the bacteria.

The first indications of suffering from swimmer's ear are a general blocked-up feeling accompanied by itching. As the symptoms continue to develop, the ear canal becomes swollen and a thin milky discharge may appear. With full-blown swimmer's ear, the sufferer will feel pain and the ear will be sensitive to the touch, particularly the cartilage in front of the ear canal.

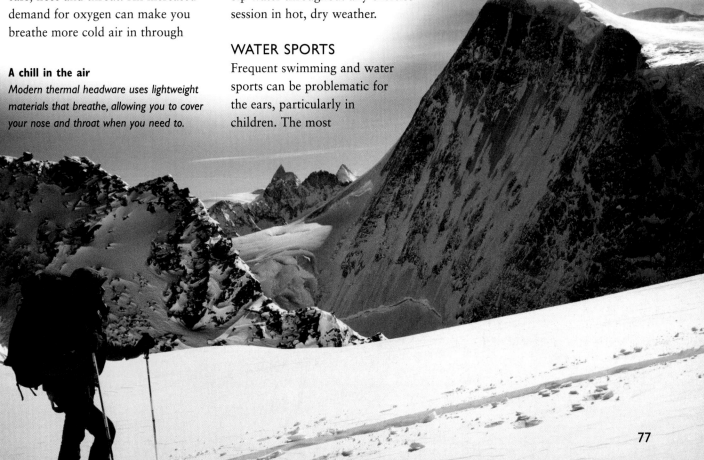

TALKING
POINT

Are nose dilator strips effective?

Nose dilator strips have become almost ubiquitous throughout the world of sport, especially among football players. The theory is that they make breathing easier by widening the nostrils, but their effectiveness has not been scientifically proven. In fact, it seems more likely that proper breathing techniques are responsible for improved performance, but the psychological effect of wearing these strips should not be underestimated. They have become so common that athletes who do not wear them may feel at a disadvantage to those who do.

Pools and your health

It is important to remember that although chlorine kills many bacteria and viruses, it does not sterilise a swimming pool. In very hot weather, chlorine is less stable and greater numbers of people are likely to be using a swimming pool. Infections of the nose and ears, as well as of the eyes if you are not wearing goggles, can all be passed on.

EQUALISING THE PRESSURE

Scuba diving (scuba stands for 'self-contained underwater breathing apparatus') allows you to go far deeper into water than unassisted diving. The deeper you go, the greater the pressure of the water environment, the effects of which are felt mostly by the ears. As your body tries to adjust to the changing pressure, you will feel an increasing need to make your ears pop or to 'equalise' (see page 62). An inability

to do so should be taken very seriously since the result could be a ruptured eardrum. This is particularly likely in divers suffering from a cold or an allergy.

CONTACT SPORTS

Activities such as boxing and rugby and other contact sports can be hazardous for the ears and nose. While the practice at turning and moving undoubtedly helps balance and coordination, boxers and rugby players suffer more broken noses and deformed, or cauliflower, ears than any other groups of sportspeople. If you are intending to box or play rugby or any other contact sport, use every safety protection available and get any injury attended to as a medical emergency.

If you have suffered any injury to your nose and ears, avoid all contact sports, including football, until given the go-ahead by your doctor.

If you develop swimmer's ear you should stop swimming and consult a doctor. You may be prescribed antibiotics or eardrops to clear up the infection, or it may be best resolved with time. Be careful not to get any water in your ears either during bathing or showering, for as long as the infection lasts.

When you do resume swimming, be cautious of how much water gets into the ear. Wearing earplugs can help, so ask your pharmacist or pool attendant for advice on the most suitable type for you. Finally, dry your ears thoroughly after swimming – to do this either shake your head gently from side to side to remove the water, or use alcohol ear drops (available from pharmacies). These evaporate excess water.

Self protection
Many rugby players protect the head with a strong helmet: this should reduce the incidence of cauliflower ear among players, and helps to avert potential brain damage.

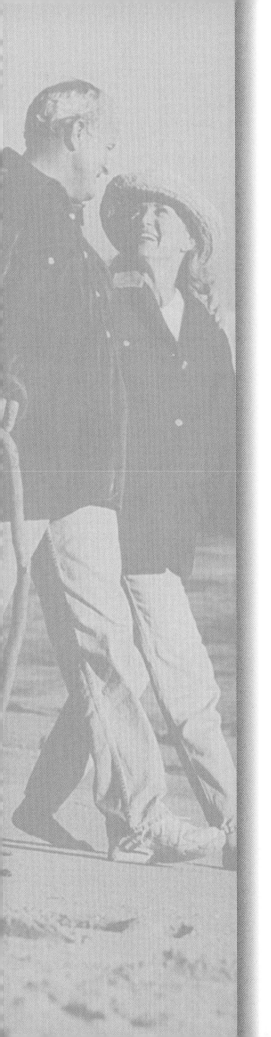

ENVIRONMENTAL RISK FACTORS

Every day, in our homes and workplaces, and in the outside atmosphere, substances that are potentially harmful to the ears, nose and throat abound. Knowing the risks and taking sensible precautions can go a long way to keeping these parts of the body healthy and functioning well.

80 *Noise is not only one of life's biggest stressors – it can also seriously damage hearing. Learn how to minimise the risks.*

85 *Being aware of the pollutants that are in every breath that meets your nose and throat is an important step to health.*

87 *Even our homes can compromise our health – discover ways to avoid the majority of household ENT irritants.*

91 *Even if you suffer from allergies, gardening need not be off limits if you take some simple precautions and choose your time.*

Noise pollution

Because the damage that is done to hearing is invisible, and often only detected years later, we tend not to notice that it is being harmed. It is a fact, however, that hearing is easy to damage, both instantly and in the long term.

The human auditory system has evolved over millions of years to allow humans to extract the maximum amount of useful information from the environment, and this is all entirely beneficial. As in many other fields, however, industrial progress has brought with it a number of problems, including:

- The risk of occupational hearing loss for people working in industrial situations which are so noisy that normal speech and other natural sounds are drowned out.
- An ability to create louder and louder sounds, through advances in amplification technology.

- The risk of severe annoyance, sleep disturbance and psychological stress for people living near to main roads, airports, railways, industrial and commercial sites, as well as those who have inconsiderate neighbours.

We all need to be aware of these risks, but we should not get them out of proportion.

GOOD SOUND, BAD SOUND

For most people most of the time, the sounds around them are cause for celebration – life would be infinitely less rewarding if we couldn't hear speech, music and the sounds of nature. However, sound does have properties which, in excess, can damage human hearing.

Sound waves

Sound consists of vibrating waves that reach the ears. These waves have two essential characteristics: amplitude, which is the loudness or volume of a sound; and frequency, which is its pitch.

Only 15 minutes exposure a day to the noise level of a rock concert can damage hearing.

In order for your ear to detect sound waves, their volume must be high enough to move the eardrum – inside which are the tiny bones that convert the sound waves into mechanical vibrations, which are then converted to nerve impulses by the stereocilia and sent to the brain for interpretation (see page 24).

From safe to harmful
The human ear can pick up an incredible range of volumes. The lowest sound level on the decibel scale (dB), 0dB, is the level of the quietest sound pressure that anybody with so-called normal hearing can hear. Continuous exposure to sounds of 85–90dB and more can damage hearing.

60 to 65dB – normal conversational speech at around 1m distance

80dB – loud music from the radio

90dB – motorcycle; rush-hour city traffic

95dB – chainsaw in operation

100–110dB – small firecrackers; thunderstorm

On the other hand, the noise must not be so loud that it perforates the eardrum or damages the stereocilia.

For your ears to pick up sound waves, not only do the waves have to be a certain volume, they must also be within a range of frequency that is capable of stimulating the stereocilia in the cochlea. The extent of the human hearing range is 20 to 20,000 hertz (Hz), but different people are sensitive to different frequencies.

NOISE AND YOUR HEALTH

Sound can be dangerous to the human body in two ways. Firstly, loud noise has the potential to cause physical damage to the ear that can result in hearing problems. Secondly, prolonged noise can produce emotional distress. Most people would agree that noise pollution is at best extremely annoying and at worst painful to the ear. Although the evidence is inconclusive, it seems that it may also have an impact on your health.

Physical damage

Loud noise is one of your ears' greatest enemies. The ears are extremely sensitive and damage to any part of their structure can cause problems. Such damage is caused by either prolonged exposure to a loud noise or by a sudden instance of noise. Damage can be permanent or temporary, and repeated instances of temporary harm may add up to permanent damage. Damage to the ears doesn't necessarily mean hearing loss: ringing in the ears and physical or psychological sensitivity to some sounds are also classed as ear damage.

- **Tinnitus** Tinnitus is a persistent ringing in the ears which can be caused by very loud noise such as that at a disco or rock concert. Usually in these instances tinnitus only lasts a few hours and normal hearing then returns, but it can be an on-going condition. It also causes hyperacusis, an extreme sensitivity to sound, in about 40 per cent of tinnitus sufferers.

What is a decibel?

A decibel is a measure of the intensity of sound, expressed as power per unit surface area. The scale starts on the threshold of human hearing, 0dB, and extends upward. The threshold of pain is about 120–140dB. Like the Richter scale which measures earthquakes, the decibel scale is logarithmic, with a base of 10. This means is that 10dB is 10 times louder than 0dB; 20dB is 10 times louder than 10dB (10x10) and 30dB is 10 times louder than 20dB (10x10x10).

Tinnitus is common in people with hearing loss, but people with 'normal' hearing can also suffer from tinnitus.

- **Temporary hearing loss** This is the feeling of slight deafness you feel when you leave a rock concert, for

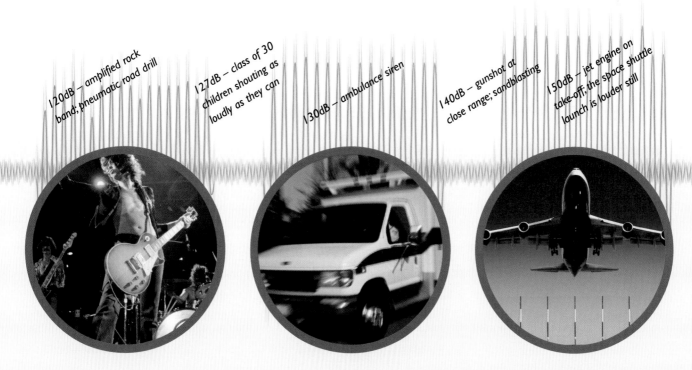

120dB – amplified rock band; pneumatic road drill

127dB – class of 30 children shouting as loudly as they can

130dB – ambulance siren

140dB – gunshot at close range; sandblasting

150dB – jet engine on take-off; the space shuttle launch is louder still

example. Your hearing will recover from this trauma, but when it does depends on how long you were listening and how loud the music was.

- **Permanent hearing loss** Permanent hearing loss may be gradual, caused by exposure to noise over a period of time. This is sometimes referred to as occupational hearing loss. Like age-related hearing loss, it initially occurs in only a narrow band of frequencies, which widens with repeated exposure. Acoustic trauma is the instant loss of hearing caused by a short, very loud noise. This type of hearing loss is often more pronounced in the ear closest to the noise, which can affect your ability to perceive sounds, or your ability to analyse sounds reaching the ears.

HOW NOISY IS TOO NOISY?

The Royal National Institute for Deaf People (RNID) gives the following guidelines for judging whether a sound is too loud.

- If you cannot talk to people about two metres away without shouting because of background noise, noise levels are dangerous.
- If you have ever been to a club or concert and found you cannot hear well for a few hours afterwards, or if you have had ringing in your ears, the sound was loud enough to damage your ears. You may have a slight, but permanent, hearing loss.
- If the level of a sound hurts your ears, you need to protect them immediately or leave the source.

The RNID advise that sounds over 80dB have the potential to damage your ears. This is about the decibel level of shouting.

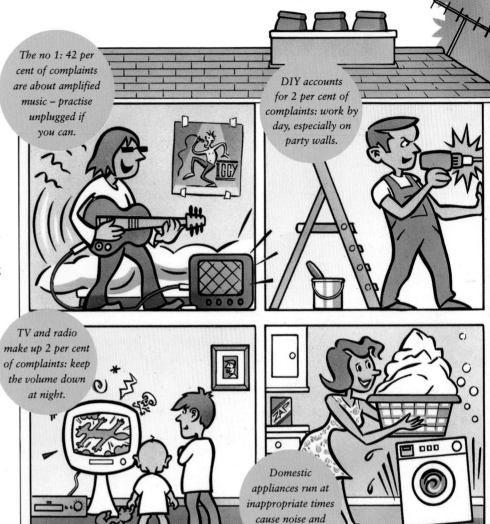

The no 1: 42 per cent of complaints are about amplified music – practise unplugged if you can.

DIY accounts for 2 per cent of complaints: work by day, especially on party walls.

TV and radio make up 2 per cent of complaints: keep the volume down at night.

Domestic appliances run at inappropriate times cause noise and vibration.

PSYCHOLOGICAL STRESS

Several factors, including sleep disturbance, anger and modified social behaviour, have been attributed to noise pollution.

Stressed out

Your body responds automatically to noise in various ways. Most of these responses are completely normal and not necessarily harmful. People who are continually exposed to potentially threatening noises adapt to them, but may start to anticipate them. In theory at least, in susceptible individuals, this can lead to a chronic build-up of stress hormones and psychological anxiety. This has an impact on quality of life and may adversely affect an individual's long-term health.

Noisy nights

Evidence suggests that most people adapt to noise at night or at least change their behaviour to compensate in some way. Electroencephalogram (EEG) measurements show harmless neural responses to familiar noises while the subject is asleep, only a small proportion of which go on to cause any measurable disruption to the normal pattern of sleep. This might be a change from a deeper to a lighter stage of sleep, sometimes even leading to awakening, but contrary to the general impression given by complaints about sleep disturbance caused by noise, it is remarkable how few noise events actually cause any measurable or significant disruption. Problems occur when

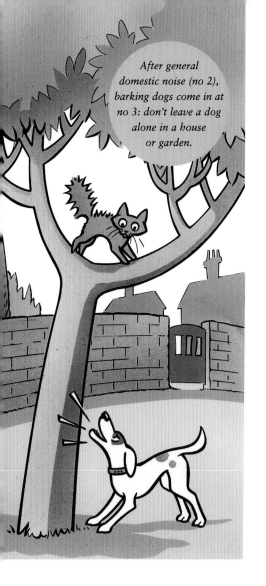

After general domestic noise (no 2), barking dogs come in at no 3: don't leave a dog alone in a house or garden.

Noisy neighbours
Local authorities publish tables of 'noisy neighbour' complaints received. Almost all sources of irritating noise can be avoided.

the noise is particularly loud or unexpected (such as a sudden thunderstorm), intermittent or unfamiliar to your brain.

There may, in addition, be individuals who cannot help anticipating the noise, thereby magnifying their anxiety and response. This can cause wakefulness and even sleep deprivation, which has an adverse effect on health.

WHAT YOU CAN DO
Minimising noise pollution can be difficult, particularly in the instance of acoustic trauma, since loud noises are often impossible to predict, so you cannot take steps to protect yourself. Despite this, the key to looking after your ears, and reducing noise-related stress, is to understand when you are in damaging environments and either alleviate the source, or take protective measures.

At home
Although our homes are quieter than the outside world, there are still steps you can take to protect your ears.
- **TV, radio and sound systems** Keep noise to a reasonable level: you should be able to talk easily over any piece of equipment. Be careful of the volume coming out of headphones, and that in confined spaces like your car. This also helps neighbourly relations.
- **DIY** If you are using noisy equipment make sure you wear ear protection. This also applies to using garden equipment.
- **Sports and leisure** Your hobbies may be putting your ears at risk. Anyone who rides a motorbike or goes clay pigeon shooting should wear ear protection.

At work
Not all jobs are located in obviously noisy environments, but it pays to be vigilant. Noise levels in restaurant kitchens, for example, can be high at busy times, and workers in call centres may be exposed to loud noise through their headsets, if these have not been fitted with loudness limiting devices.
- **Machinery** Workplaces with machinery operating are usually among the loudest. Garages, factories, construction sites and road works are obvious examples. Agricultural workers and horticulturists may also be at risk.
- **Music** Consider noise levels if you work in an environment where

---

FOR THE UNDER 12s

Children and noise

Two recent studies have looked at the effect of airport noise on children. In Munich, Germany, more than 200 children were tested for blood pressure and levels of stress hormones six months before, and six months after, the opening of a new international airport. The second study looked at children living near the JFK international airport in New York.

Although the results were not wholly conclusive in either test, children who lived under the flight path in Munich were shown to have higher blood pressure and levels of stress hormones than those who did not. (The two groups of children were matched in terms of other factors, such as age, parental occupation and socio-economic status.)

Higher blood pressure and levels of stress hormones may be related to heart problems and raised cholesterol in adulthood. The New York study found some evidence that children near the airport did not read or listen as well as children from other areas of the city.

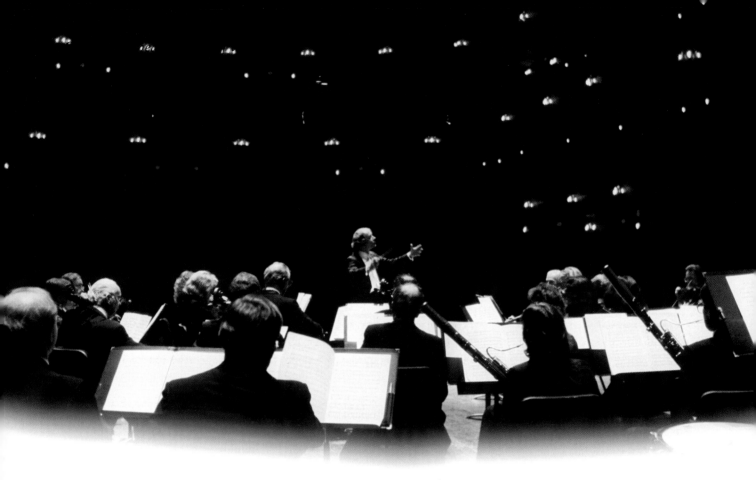

Musical chairs

Musicians may suffer trauma to the ears if seated too close to the noisiest instruments, often the brass and percussion sections. While earplugs may be available, some musicians find playing while wearing them is not easy.

music is permanently playing, such as record stores, some bars and sports centres.

• Transport Jet engines are among the biggest noise makers, so airport workers must be especially vigilant. All city traffic contributes to noise levels, so anyone who works in city streets should take care.

Employers are legally required to protect you when you are at work, and this includes your hearing. Your employer should have practices in place to assess the level of noise in all areas. If this level exceeds 85dB, you should be alerted to the risks to your hearing, noisy areas should be clearly marked with warning signs, and you should be provided with protection for your ears. If you work

in a noisy environment, employers are required to have your hearing tested and monitored by experts.

Employees have responsibilities, too, however. Everyone should evaluate their individual exposure to noise, and if necessary take precautions. Failing to protect your ears if you work for extended periods in a noisy environment will cause cumulative permanent damage. This will also happen if your ear protection doesn't fit properly: check this by listening to your voice, which should sound louder and deeper if your protection is working properly. Short breaks are also beneficial.

Out and about

It is almost impossible to predict noises in the environment, but being aware of the risk may help you to minimise exposure. Be sure to wear earplugs at rock concerts and in music clubs. If a cinema soundtrack hurts your ears, ask if it can be turned down. If not, leave.

What ear protection is available?

Two types of headgear protect the eardrums – earmuffs and earplugs. Both decrease the volume of sound allowed to reach your middle ear, by sealing off the ear canal. Whether you choose earmuffs or earplugs, they will only be of use if they fit properly, and so reduce noise by 15 to 30dB. Good quality earplugs and earmuffs offer approximately equal sound reductions, although earplugs are considered better for low frequency noise and earmuffs for high frequency noise. Using both types of protection at once will reduce noise by a further 10 to 15dB and should be considered in high-risk areas.

ASK THE EXPERT

Knowing the atmospheric irritants

Atmospheric pollution is all around us – in our homes, in workplaces and in the outdoor environment. Increasing concentrations may mean that your nose and throat need a helping hand to defend themselves.

The environment is full of chemicals and gases, as well as more naturally occurring irritants. Symptoms that are slow to clear, such as a stuffy head, itchy throat or runny nose, may be an indication of atmospheric irritants in your environment.

TYPES OF POLLUTION

There are two main types of airborne irritants that can adversely affect your health:

- Toxic air pollutants, including gases and vapours such as carbon monoxide, as well as petrochemical fumes, for example from household cleaning products
- Particulate matter, including dust and dust mites, and pollen from trees, shrubs and flowers

When you breathe in these airborne pollutants they can cause a number of temporary ailments. Most – including a runny nose and itchy throat – occur in the nose and throat. In many cases these symptoms are temporary, but they may signal potential long-term damage being done to the body. Just as even the best sieve on the market lets some impurities into your cooking, so the nose cannot filter out 100 per cent of pollutants, particularly when the particles or atoms are too small to be trapped.

Toxic airborne pollutants can be poisonous in small or large doses, instantly and over time.

TOXIC AIR POLLUTANTS

There are many sources of toxic pollutants in the environment. A number irritate the nose and throat, and all increase your risk of lung or bronchial disease, paralysis or fits. These fall into two groups: gases, vapours and fumes; and petrochemicals. These groupings make them easier to identify in, and eventually eradicate from, your environment (see pages 88–89 for tips on a healthy home).

- **Gases, vapours and fumes** Gases such as carbon monoxide are exceedingly dangerous at high levels. Other harmful gases include carbon dioxide, nitric oxide and sulphur dioxide. These may irritate your nose and throat, but their main damage is to the lungs, where they can severely impede breathing and cause respiratory paralysis.

Fresh country air?
Most people assume that country air is less polluted than city air. This is largely true, but there are still risks that must be controlled, such as spraying of agricultural chemicals.

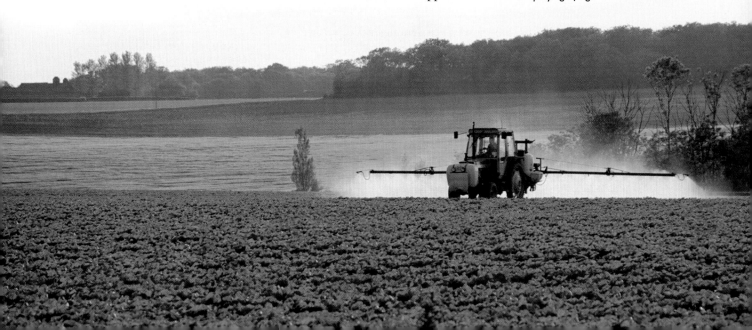

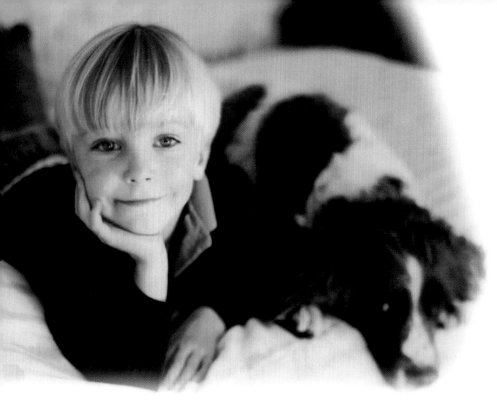

Pets and allergies
Recent studies suggest that pets may not always be off limits for children with allergies. One study which followed children from birth to the age of seven found that those born into a household where there was already a cat or dog were less likely to suffer allergies than other children.

• Petrochemicals Petrochemicals are organic compounds found in many manufactured products. They can become dangerous if fumes accumulate, and can affect the mucous membranes in the eyes, mouth, throat and lungs. They also increase the risk of cancer.

PARTICULATE MATTER

Particulate matter irritates the nose and throat. This is not only because these body parts are in charge of filtering out airborne particles, it is also due to the allergic reactions such particles can trigger.

> *85 per cent of children who experience allergic asthma are sensitive to house-dust mites.*

Symptoms of an allergic reaction include sneezing, a runny or stuffy nose, watery and itchy eyes and possibly headaches. Some allergies can also trigger asthma. Those who suffer from allergies are often sensitive to quite a number of allergens, and some of the most common are dust, pet hair and dander, and mould.

The demon dust and dust mites

Dust is not just dirt and grime, it includes a mixture of particles of skin, pet hair, food, clothing and furnishings. Dust also contains microscopic dust mites that thrive in the warm, humid conditions found in modern buildings. It is mainly the faecal pellets of these dust mites that trigger the allergic reactions that cause respiratory problems, including asthma and inflammation of the mucous membranes. Dust mites live in upholstery, carpets and bedding.

Pollen

The seasonal type of allergic rhinitis is called hay fever, and is most commonly caused by a reaction to pollen released by grasses, flowers and trees. Pollen are the microscopic grains that plants manufacture to reproduce. Certain types of pollen are small, dry, light grains that travel very effectively on the air. It is predominantly these types that are referred to as atmospheric irritants, and that play havoc with the sinuses of hay fever sufferers.

Mould is also something to watch out for in the garden. Both the mould itself and the spores it produces can cause allergic rhinitis.

Treatments

The most common treatment for allergic rhinitis is the prescription of anti-histamine tablets, as well as the use of cortisone inhalers and nasal sprays to help reduce inflammation and swelling. Alternative therapies are also popular with allergy sufferers (see pages 57–58). The most effective remedy, however, is to reduce the number of airborne irritants in your environment.

What is allergic rhinitis?

Allergic rhinitis occurs when your immune system over-reacts to a foreign substance that does not bother most people, such as pollen or dust. In such cases the body manufactures elevated levels of an antibody called immunoglobulin E (IgE). Each IgE antibody binds to a specific allergen. When the two bind together, they stimulate the body's mast cells to release strong inflammatory chemicals, such as histamine.

ASK THE EXPERT

A healthy home and garden

Our homes and gardens are our last refuge from the stresses of the world, but they are not always safe havens. Both indoor and outdoor air can be polluted and may have a serious impact on your nose and throat.

INDOOR AIR QUALITY

Creating a home that is relatively free of airborne pollutants takes effort, but with time and care you will soon notice an improvement in the symptoms of exposure to atmospheric irritants, such as runny nose, sneezing and sore throat.

GAS, VAPOUR AND FUME-FREE LIVING

It is important to eliminate or reduce fumes and toxic gases. To do this, check the services coming into the building for leaks, especially gas pipes. If you have a choice, build a garage separate from the house, or keep the connecting door to the house closed so that exhaust fumes do not get into the house. Check that gas from cookers and heaters is properly vented to the outside – never use a gas heater in a closed room. When buying a new fireplace or restoring an old one, install a sealed primary or secondary combustion stove. These are energy efficient and environment-friendly.

Eliminating petrochemicals

Petrochemicals give off fumes into the air and are found in an enormous number of products in our homes. Synthetic carpets and underlay, in particular, are laden with them. To reduce petrochemical fumes, replace your carpet with floorboards or coverings made from natural fibres such as wool, jute, sea grass or coir. The furnishings and fabrics in your home may also have been chemically treated and can emit fumes. The best replacements for these materials are organic natural fibres that have not been bleached or treated, including linen, hessian or cotton.

Many chemical irritants are found in ordinary household cleaners, especially those for ovens, carpets, windows and upholstery. Formaldehyde, phenols, ammonia and chlorine are found in bleaches, disinfectants, detergents, air fresheners and personal hygiene products and have all been found to increase health risks. Symptoms include inflammation of mucous membranes, nasal congestion, upper respirator tract infection, nausea, headache and eye irritation.

What are the irritants?

When purchasing products, read the labels to see what you are getting. If you can't avoid irritant chemicals, be careful not to breathe in their fumes.

ACETONE (nail polish remover)
nose, throat, eye and lung irritation, headaches, dizziness

AMMONIA (household cleaners)
breathing problems

BENZENE (dyes, detergents)
headache, dizziness, nausea and breathing difficulties

ETHYL ALCOHOL (antifreeze)
eye irritation, breathing difficulties, headache, drowsiness

ETHYL ACETATE (printing inks)
anaemia, eye, nose and gum irritations, breathing difficulties, lethargy

FORMALDEHYDE (fibreboards)
breathing difficulties, eye, ear and nose irritation

METHYL ALCOHOL (solvents)
headache, nausea, irritation of mucous membranes

TOLUENE (paint, paint thinners)
impaired co-ordination, mental sluggishness, loss of hearing and vision

TRICHLOROETHYLENE (degreasers)
headaches, dizziness, memory loss, breathing difficulties

XYLENE (paint, paint thinners)
nausea, cough, inflammation of mucous membranes, nose and throat irritation

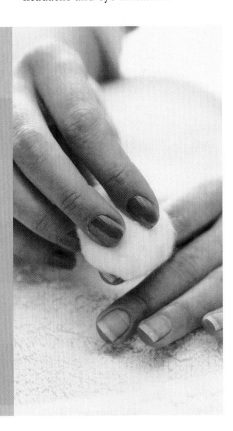

KEEPING MITES AT BAY

House-dust mites are inevitable in today's homes. They provoke irritation of the nasal passages and eyes, and are the major cause of asthma symptoms in many sufferers. Controlling the number of them in your home needs a regular and methodical approach. Here are eight tips to get you started:

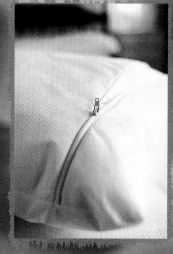

PROTECT YOUR BEDDING
Cover your mattress, duvet and pillows with a dust mite-proof barrier cover.

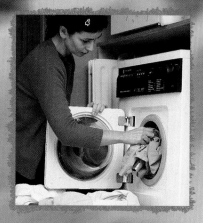

HOT-WASH BEDDING
Washing bed covers, sheets and pillow cases at 60°C removes mites and their droppings.

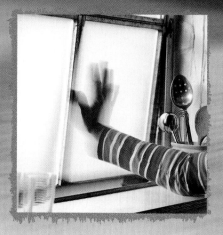

VENTILATE
Thoroughly ventilating the house, by opening the windows, helps to prevent damp.

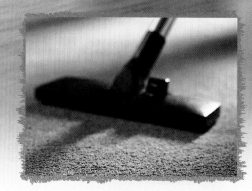

VACUUM REGULARLY
Vacuuming daily with an efficient vacuum cleaner and damp dusting picks up mites and their droppings.

MAKE YOUR HOME A DUST-FREE ZONE

It is unrealistic to expect to be able to get rid of all airborne irritants in our homes, but we can do a great deal to reduce dust. Living in a dust-free zone will have a dramatic effect on your health, even if you do not suffer from allergies or asthma.

Remove clutter from window-sills and tabletops, especially ornaments, picture frames, books and magazines which collect a great deal of dust. Open the windows and thoroughly air your home and then dust all surfaces well. It is a good idea to use an electrostatically charged cloth, which will pick up the dust without re-releasing it into the air.

Wash your curtains and loose soft furnishings using a detergent made from natural products. Vertical blinds will collect less dust than traditional curtains, swags and drapes or venetian blinds.

Carpets hold and release dust. If you are keen to retain carpet, replace synthetic carpets and underlay with those made from natural fibres. Vacuum them well and, if possible, get them steam-cleaned using eco-friendly products that do not contain chemical irritants. Ideally, you should replace carpets with a solid floor covering. The more flat, even and smooth floor surfaces you have in your home, the less opportunity there is for dust to build up. For this

IT'S NOT TRUE!

'Short-haired breeds do not cause allergies'

The problem with hairy or furry pets is not their hair or fur. It is their dander, microscopic particles of dead skin, and saliva which provoke symptoms. Despite evidence to the contrary from asthma sufferers, research has shown that short-haired pets are as much of a problem as long-haired ones. Even hairless breeds can provoke asthma symptoms or allergic reactions.

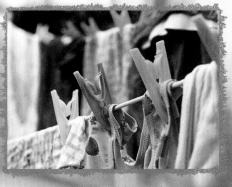

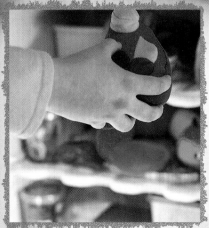

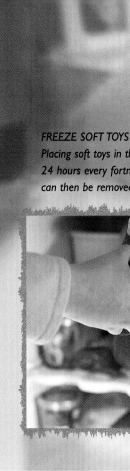

FREEZE SOFT TOYS
Placing soft toys in the freezer for 24 hours every fortnight kills mites, which can then be removed by hot-washing.

PREVENT STATIC
Dry your clothing and washing outside whenever possible (unless you suffer from hay fever).

AIR BEDDING
Air your bedding regularly, especially in winter when homes tend to be less well ventilated.

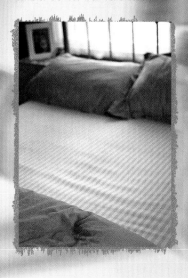

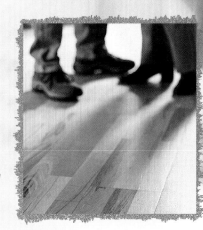

PREVENT DUST BUILD-UP
Replace carpets with a smooth-finish timber or other even floor surface, such as vinyl.

There are more than two million house-dust mites in the average double mattress.

reason smooth timber floors are recommended for anyone who regularly suffers from asthma or other allergies.

Vacuum frequently, especially where there is carpet. If your machine has a filter, make sure you change it regularly, and if any member of the household is particularly sensitive to dust you could consider buying a vacuum cleaner fitted with high efficiency particulate air (HEPA) filters.

Do not allow pets into bedrooms as some of their allergens are carried on very small particles and will remain airborne for long periods.

Pet dander is difficult to remove from carpets and furnishings and easily transfers onto clothes. Restricting your pet's access inside the house will dramatically reduce the level of allergen exposure. You can further minimise the problem by having your pet regularly washed and groomed. If anyone in your home keeps rabbits, rats, guinea pigs or gerbils, keep these in a secure hutch away from the house.

Desensitisation treatment may have benefits, so it is worth discussing this option with your specialist.

OTHER MEANS AND METHODS

In addition to reducing the pollutants and irritants that enter your home, there is plenty you can do to minimise the impact of substances that are already present and are difficult to eliminate.

Ventilation

While it is only natural to want to be warm and dry in the home in winter, lack of proper ventilation can cause health problems. Like you, your house needs to breathe, and it does this through the walls as well as through doors and windows. Dust and pollution soon build up inside a sealed house. Damp and humid

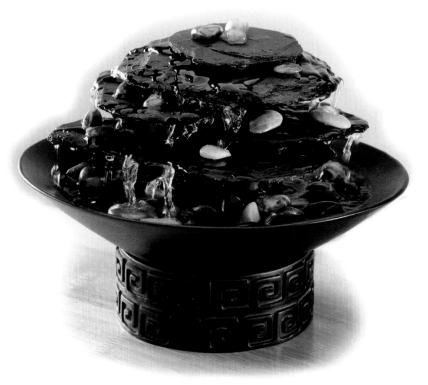

Water feature

If you do not want to buy an ioniser, there is a natural alternative. Moving water creates negative ions, and so by introducing a small indoor water feature or pebble fountain into your home, the air will be naturally ionised.

What does an ioniser do?

In a natural clean outdoor environment the electrostatic balance of positive and negative ions in the air is approximately equal. Inside a building, however, the negative ions are depleted by many facets of daily living, such as breathing, heating, air conditioning and computers. This imbalance causes the positively charged ions to attract and hold dust particles and can cause various health problems, including allergies. An ioniser works to restore electrical balance.

ASK THE EXPERT

conditions encourage mould to form, and create an environment in which house-dust mites flourish. If your house feels damp, check for leaks as well as rising damp. It may be that moisture is trapped inside a cavity wall, in which case you will need professional advice on what you can do to help it escape so that your house can dry out. Removing leaks and rising damp from your home can be a tall order.

Most modern homes are finished with non-porous paints, which trap moisture inside. A dehumidifier can regulate excess moisture but does not necessarily solve the problem. One solution is to strip non-porous paint and re-paint the inside and outside of your house with porous paint which allows the water inside to evaporate into the air outside.

Air conditioning

Air conditioning systems contain filters that reduce the number of airborne pollutants brought into the home from outside. Air conditioning also reduces the humidity in the air it circulates, which cuts down on potential moulds and fungi. However, poor maintenance leads to a less efficient system, and can provide a perfect breeding ground for airborne diseases that may then be distributed throughout the air-conditioned environment.

Air filters

When choosing an air filter, you should make sure that it is a HEPA (high efficiency particulate air) filter, and keep in mind that the greater the surface area of the filter the more effectively it will work. Such filters have been shown to benefit asthmatics and allergy sufferers, and are often combined with an activated carbon filter to clear chemical pollution from the air.

Electrostatic filters

These are generally useful in filtering smoke and other larger particulate matter, but are less effective for smaller particles such as airborne bacteria and viruses, and gases and odours. This restricts their usefulness to allergy sufferers.

Air ionisers

Simple ionisers draw in air and give dust particles a negative charge so that dirt is attracted out of the air and onto the nearest relatively positively charged surface, from which it can easily be cleaned. Electrostatic filters also ionise air passing through them but contain a positively charged filter to collect the dust particles as they pass through the device, resulting in cleaner air.

There is evidence, however, that ionisers can increase some symptoms, such as night-time cough.

When springtime isn't fun

During the onset of spring and its progression through to summer, there is a general pattern to the order in which species pollinate. This pattern can help sufferers to avoid certain triggers.

A HEALTHY GARDEN

Although you can't eliminate all the airborne pollutants from the outdoor environment, you can significantly reduce their concentration in your own garden.

GARDEN IRRITANTS

Two of the biggest garden irritants to your nose and throat are pollen from trees, flowers, grass and weeds, and spores from moulds and fungi growing in rotting vegetation.

Mould spores are the reproductive particles of mould. Each spore can give rise to a new mould that can produce millions more spores. Both the spores and tiny fragments of mould can cause allergic rhinitis if they are inhaled.

People who suffer from allergic rhinitis (hay fever) are sensitive to pollen and moulds and can have acute symptoms including a runny or stuffy nose, inflammation of the nose and throat, irritation of the eyes and inflammation of the sinuses.

IF YOU HAVE ALLERGIES

Carefully monitoring pollen levels, taking preventive and protective measures, and avoiding plants that release pollen into the air can minimise problems and let you enjoy your garden.

Pollen levels

Pollen levels are widely monitored and the European Aeroallergen Network coordinates information

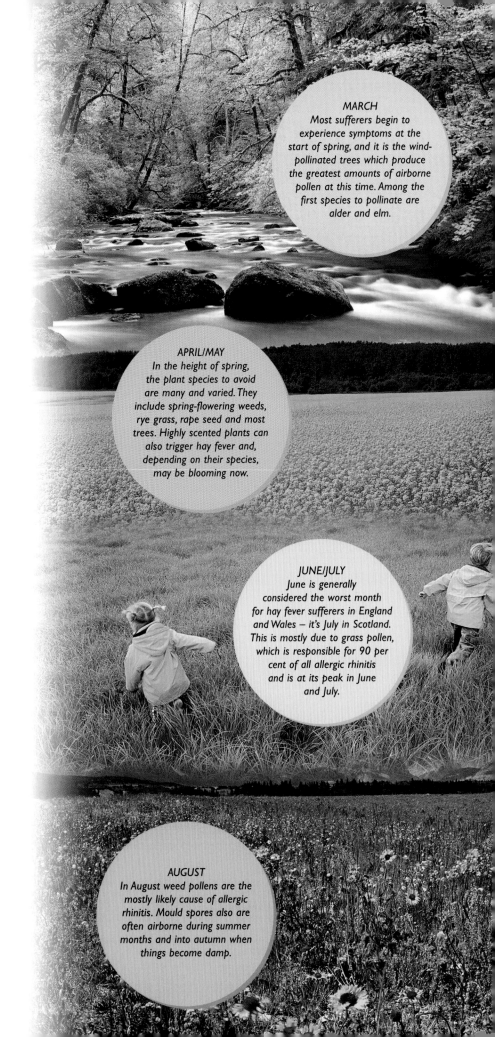

MARCH
Most sufferers begin to experience symptoms at the start of spring, and it is the wind-pollinated trees which produce the greatest amounts of airborne pollen at this time. Among the first species to pollinate are alder and elm.

APRIL/MAY
In the height of spring, the plant species to avoid are many and varied. They include spring-flowering weeds, rye grass, rape seed and most trees. Highly scented plants can also trigger hay fever and, depending on their species, may be blooming now.

JUNE/JULY
June is generally considered the worst month for hay fever sufferers in England and Wales – it's July in Scotland. This is mostly due to grass pollen, which is responsible for 90 per cent of all allergic rhinitis and is at its peak in June and July.

AUGUST
In August weed pollens are the mostly likely cause of allergic rhinitis. Mould spores also are often airborne during summer months and into autumn when things become damp.

on major allergens from monitoring stations throughout Europe. Daily weather reports, and information on Teletext and Ceefax also give warnings of high pollen levels. When levels are expected to be exceptionally high remain indoors if possible. Keep an eye on local weather conditions, too, and use them to your benefit.

- Early morning rain prevents the release of pollen that day so any allergy should not be a problem on those days; rain later in the day washes pollen from the air.
- Wind stirs up pollen and dust so take every precaution on blustery days; similarly on hot, still days pollen 'hangs' in the air.

Does wearing a mask protect my nose from pollen?

Wearing a facemask on days when the pollen count is high can drastically reduce the irritating particles entering your nose, as long as you follow instructions on changing and cleaning the filter. The best types of mask are those made from an electrostatically charged material that filters out very small particles down to 0.04 of a micron. This gives much better protection than an ordinary facemask, which only filters out larger particles. A scarf or handkerchief will provide hardly any protection at all, as the pollen and dust particles are small enough to pass through the weave of the fabric.

ASK THE EXPERT

- Sunny days raise pollen to cloud level during the morning, and it only falls when the temperature starts to drop. Do any gardening in the early morning or afternoon, or restrict it to cool, cloudy days.

Cutting the lawn

It is best to cut the lawn in the early morning, ideally while there is still a little dew to dampen things down. Regular trimming is a good idea, and it is better to use a cylinder or rotary mower rather than an electric powered one, to restrict blowing the grass cuttings around (a machine with a box to collect the clippings is best). Close the windows of the house before and for some time after.

All gardeners with allergies must pay careful attention to their clothes. Wear a long-sleeved shirt, hat, gloves and dark glasses to avoid eye and skin contact with plants that could cause an allergic reaction. A purpose-made mask is useful. After being outdoors, shower to wash off the pollen that will have collected on your clothes, body and in your hair. Don't wear your gardening clothes in the house.

Weeding

Hoeing is more sensible than weeding, if you can keep weeds under control in this way, as your nose and eyes are further away from the plants. Planting good ground-cover can reduce or even eliminate the need for weeding. Low-allergen ground-cover plants which also suppress weeds include vinca (periwinkle), ajuga, campanula (Canterbury bells), hostas and ferns. Covering any unplanted areas with plastic sheeting or gravel mulch can also suppress weeds.

Choosing plants wisely

Plants vary in the amount of pollen they produce and the method they use to distribute it. Gardeners with hay fever should try to avoid wind-pollinated plants.

Wind-blown pollen is small, light and easily spread. Even if you are not allergic to pollen you could become sensitised by breathing it in, especially in large quantities. Wind-pollinated plants include all grasses, many trees, and some wild flowers. Avoid such trees as ash, birch, elder, hazel, horse chestnut, oak, plane, willow and yew.

A high-pollen tree in your garden exposes you to 10 times more pollen than a similar tree a block away.

Choose instead insect-pollinated plants, as these produce heavier, stickier pollen which is less likely to be released into the air. Most shrubs and flowers with large petals are insect pollinated, as are most herbs. Blossom trees are also generally pollinated by insects.

Try to avoid heavily scented flowers, which may trigger asthma. These include freesia, jasmine and wisteria. Even lightly scented plants can harbour wind-blown pollen, so it's best not to smell them.

The good news is that many of the brightest coloured flowers are showy precisely to attract pollinating insects, so these can form a major feature of your garden. Plants to choose include clematis, iris and violas, as well as such popular annuals as snapdragons, busy lizzies, cornflowers and love-in-a-mist.

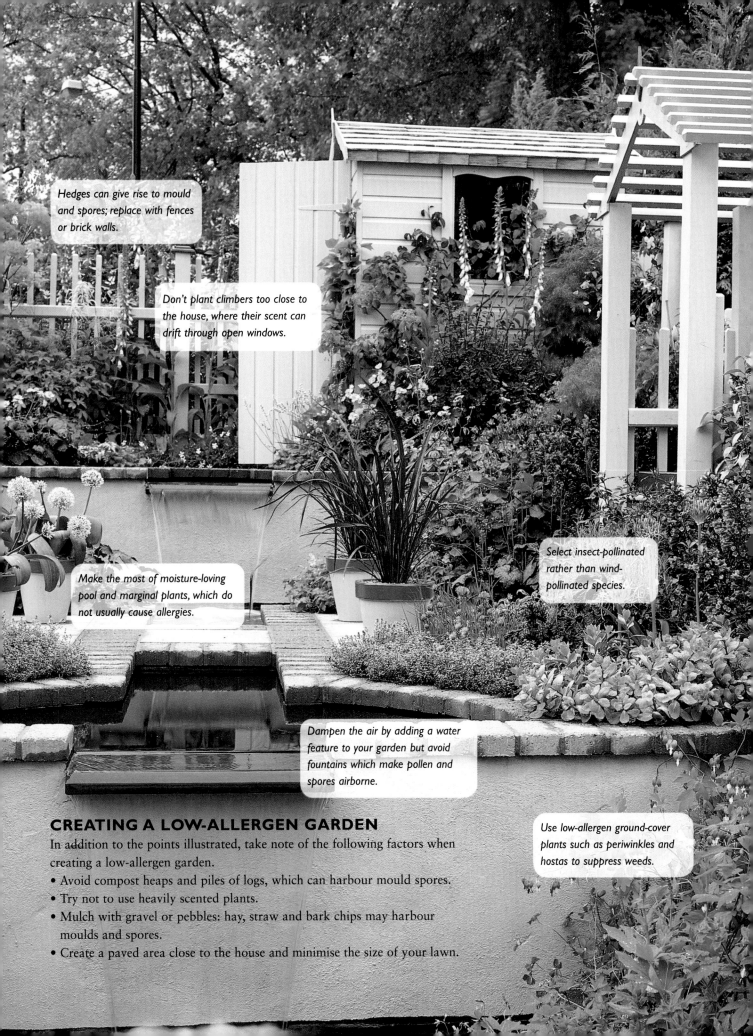

Hedges can give rise to mould and spores; replace with fences or brick walls.

Don't plant climbers too close to the house, where their scent can drift through open windows.

Make the most of moisture-loving pool and marginal plants, which do not usually cause allergies.

Select insect-pollinated rather than wind-pollinated species.

Dampen the air by adding a water feature to your garden but avoid fountains which make pollen and spores airborne.

Use low-allergen ground-cover plants such as periwinkles and hostas to suppress weeds.

CREATING A LOW-ALLERGEN GARDEN

In addition to the points illustrated, take note of the following factors when creating a low-allergen garden.

- Avoid compost heaps and piles of logs, which can harbour mould spores.
- Try not to use heavily scented plants.
- Mulch with gravel or pebbles: hay, straw and bark chips may harbour moulds and spores.
- Create a paved area close to the house and minimise the size of your lawn.

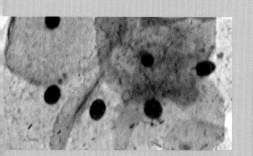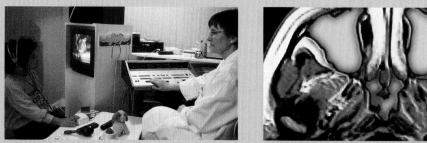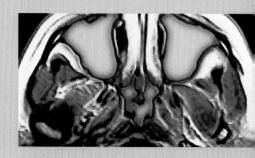

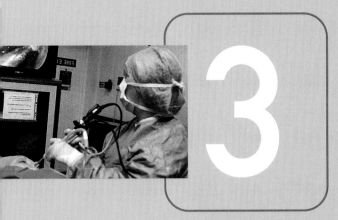

3

What happens when things go wrong

Knowing what can go wrong

Virtually everybody has had an ailment affecting the ears, nose or throat at some stage in their life. People of all ages are susceptible, and there are a number of reasons – ranging from hereditary to environmental factors – why some become ill and others do not.

Infection, injury and disease can all affect the sophisticated mechanisms of the ears, nose and throat. Recognising and understanding the various conditions and symptoms can help enormously when it comes to seeking treatment.

GENETIC AND HEREDITARY FACTORS

We all carry thousands of different genes, which give rise to the amazing diversity and variety of human beings. However, gene abnormalities may lead to a deformity that is immediately apparent at birth, or may predispose an individual to a higher chance of developing an ENT condition later in life.

Problems at birth

A specific genetic abnormality may result in a condition known as microtia, where the the external framework of the ear, or pinna, is absent or malformed at birth.

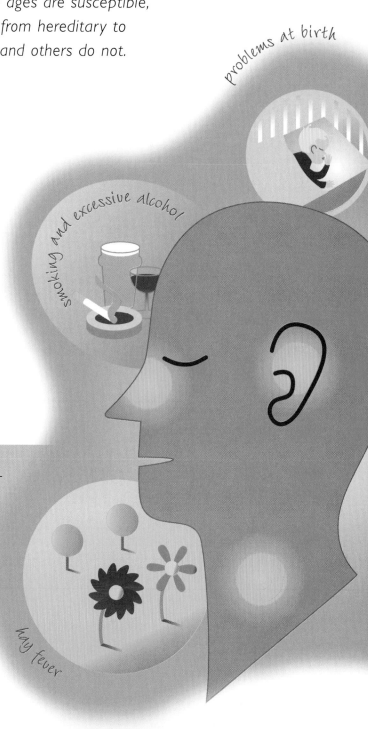

MORE COMMON

MOTION SICKNESS	TONSILLITIS/SORE THROAT
Up to 9 in 10 adults suffer from motion sickness at some time.	5524 PER 100,000 OR 1 IN 18
HEARING LOSS	HAY FEVER
1 in 5 adults have some degree of presbyacusis (age-related hearing loss); that rises to 1 in 2 of people aged over 75.	5263 PER 100,000 OR 1 IN 19

Babies with microtia are more likely to have other developmental problems of their middle and inner ears which affect their ability to hear. This may only become obvious as a child grows and starts interacting with others. Microtia is treatable: the malformed ear can be removed and a new one created from cartilage.

Some babies are predisposed to develop red vascular swellings beneath the skin called haemangiomas. When these occur in the airway they may obstruct breathing, which can be fatal. Airway haemangiomas do not typically become enlarged until several weeks after birth,

Average incidence of ENT problems
A variety of factors influence the long-term health of your ears, nose and throat. The figures above, based on UK figures for the late 1990s, show the number of people likely to contract an infection or other problem in any given year.

when they must be removed as a matter of urgency. Newborn babies may also be predominantly nose rather than mouth breathers. Narrowing of the back of the nose, known as choanal atresia, may stop them breathing effectively, leading to respiratory distress, although this can be detected and treated easily.

Problems in later life

Certain genes may make an individual more likely to develop particular types of cancer later in life, such as thyroid gland tumours. There may be no warning of the impending development of such a condition, although genetic testing of 'high-risk' individuals enables doctors to spot a problem early so that steps can be taken to reduce any other risk factors which may contribute.

ENVIRONMENTAL FACTORS

Although genetic factors may predispose an individual to the development of a particular disease, environmental factors act throughout life to influence whether or not a condition will

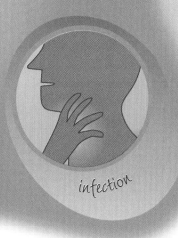

loud noise

infection

develop. Reducing or avoiding some of these environmental factors can often help to improve the chances of not developing an illness later in life.

Allergies

Many people are allergic to substances present in the atmosphere and in the home. These substances, which include pollen, house-dust mites, and animal dander

Nearly half a million operations on the ears, nose and throat were performed in the UK in 2000.

(flakes of dead skin), are known as allergens. Exposure to allergens can cause nasal congestion, sneezing and a runny nose. When reactions are triggered by tree or grass pollen during summer, the condition is known as hay fever. Treatment is based on avoidance of the allergen, together with drugs to relieve symptoms (see page 118).

Pollution

Atmospheric pollution can cause nasal congestion and rhinitis – inflammation of the nose's lining. Prolonged or highly concentrated exposure to specific occupational substances, such as nickel and hardwood shavings, is suspected of being linked to cancer of the sinuses.

Noise pollution

Noise is another form of damaging pollution. People who are regularly exposed to extreme levels of noise can suffer damage to the cochlea or labyrinth of the ear, leading to premature hearing loss.

LESS COMMON

TINNITUS	OTITIS MEDIA	GLANDULAR FEVER
4000 PER 100,000 OR 1 IN 25 HAVE PERMANENT TINNITUS TO SOME DEGREE; 1 IN 10 HAVE EXPERIENCED TINNITUS AT SOME TIME	2818 IN 100,000, OR 1 IN 35 It is mostly children who suffer from this acute ear infection.	53 per 100,000 or 1 in 1886
230,000 have tinnitus that severely effects their ability to lead a normal life.	SINUSITIS 1788 per 100,000 or 1 in 56	FAMILIAL MULTIPLE ENDOCRINE NEOPLASIA Fewer than 25 new cases of this syndrome, which can cause thyroid tumours, are reported each year.

ENT INFECTIONS

Infections are one of the most common reasons for visiting the GP, and these can affect nearly every part of the head and neck.
- **Common ear infections** include otitis media (inflammation of the middle ear) and otitis externa (inflammation of the outer ear canal).
- **Common nose infections** include rhinitis and sinusitis.
- **Common throat infections** include pharyngitis (inflammation of the throat), tonsillitis and glandular fever.

- **Common infections of the airways** include laryngitis (inflammation of the voice box) and, less commonly, tracheitis (inflammation of the windpipe).

Most of these conditions are acute, meaning that they are sudden, one-off events, after which the patient returns to good health. Chronic infections are longer-term 'grumbling' conditions that can last weeks, months or years. Environmental factors such as damp living conditions, smoking and heavy alcohol consumption can aggravate chronic infections.

TUMOURS

These can affect the ears, nose, throat and other parts of the head and neck. Tumours can be benign, that is slow growing and confined to one area of the body, or malignant, more aggressive, faster growing, and more likely to spread to other areas. Cancers may occur in the sinuses, thyroid gland, salivary glands, throat, tongue and larynx (voice box). A large number of tumours, particularly those affecting the inner lining of the nose, mouth, throat and airways, are strongly linked to smoking. Avoiding the carcinogens in tobacco greatly reduces the chance of developing these tumours.

Tumours affecting the ear, nose and throat can also appear on the skin of the head, face, neck and ears and are commonly caused by exposure to strong sunlight. These include malignant melanomas (tumours of the melanocytes, the cells that produce the skin's pigmentation) and basal cell carcinomas, also known as rodent ulcers.

PHYSICAL INJURIES

Trauma, or physical injury, is a leading cause of illness and disability, particularly in young people. Common ear injuries include a perforated eardrum and the forming of a blood clot in the ear's external cartilage. The nose may bleed if picked frequently or punched; bleeding often stops with simple pressure and ice, but is likely to persist if a larger blood vessel has been severed. Foreign bodies such as pen tops, marbles or cottonwool buds can injure the ears, nose or throat if inserted, inhaled or swallowed. Other injuries can occur during surgery; for example, vocal fold paralysis might result from damage to a laryngeal nerve during a tricky thyroidectomy.

DRUGS

Side effects of several common drugs result in problems in the ears, nose or throat. The antibiotic gentamicin, for example – often used intravenously to fight bloodstream infections – can cause profound deafness, particularly in genetically susceptible individuals. Some drugs used in the treatment of leukaemias can affect balance and hearing. The loss is not necessarily related to the dose or duration of treatment with the drug; in some cases, it occurs after one dose but can cause permanent dizziness or deafness.

LIFESTYLE

Smoking is probably the greatest single influence on whether an individual develops certain illnesses or not. Excessive alcohol consumption is also detrimental to good health, and has been linked to cancer of the mouth and tongue, especially in smokers. Although a direct link between dietary factors and the development of tumours has not been proven, experts believe that a balanced, low-fat diet with plenty of fruits and vegetables helps to maintain a healthy immune system, capable of fighting off infection and recovering from injury.

AGEING

The ageing process is responsible for a number of gradual changes that result in progressive deterioration in the functioning of some body systems. Perhaps the most common example is hearing loss. Others include increased susceptibility to infections and certain types of tumour.

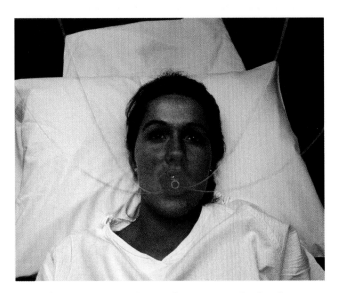

Laser-activated cancer therapy for a tumour in the throat
A low-power red argon laser passes through four optical fibre waveguides to kill cancer cells in a patient's throat by activating a drug (haematoporphyrin derivative) previously injected into the tumour.

Meet the ENT specialists

Patients with problems relating to the ears, nose and throat are usually referred to an ENT clinic. Here they will meet a wide range of specialists and technicians, who are trained to diagnose and treat all conditions of the neck and head.

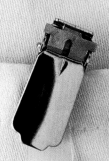

The technically correct title for the surgical speciality of ENT is otolaryngology. This term encompasses conditions of the ears, nose and throat, plus diseases of the base of the skull, head and neck, face and trachea (windpipe). Treatment can involve the use of powerful operating microscopes, fibreoptic and rigid endoscopes and lasers. The breadth of surgical skill required to meet the medical needs of patients necessitates close collaboration between ENT specialists and many other specialists, such as anaesthetic staff, neurosurgeons (who specialise in the surgical treatment of the brain and spinal cord), plastic surgeons and cardiothoracic surgeons (who specialise in the treatment of the heart and lungs).

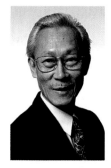

CONSULTANT OTOLARYNGOLOGIST

The consultant otolaryngologist is the head of a hospital's ENT department and is skilled in the full range of surgical disciplines, including skull base surgery, head and neck tumour surgery and airway procedures. All patients who attend an ENT clinic, or are admitted for an ENT procedure, are under the care of the consultant otolaryngologist, although most will be seen and treated by members of his or her team.

ENT NURSE

The role of the ENT nurse is to provide care for post-operative ENT patients on hospital wards. They are trained to manage and care for patients with the full range of ENT conditions. Some nurses specialise in a particular aspect of patient care. For example, tracheostomy nurse specialists are now commonplace in larger ENT units; they offer expert advice on tracheostomies and are often the first port of call for tracheostomy patients who encounter problems at home.

AUDIOLOGICAL TECHNICIAN

Many patients attending an ENT clinic require a hearing test. These are performed by audiological technicians who also prescribe and fit hearing aids, teach people how to use them effectively, and offer advice on other equipment and strategies that will help people to deal with hearing loss. In addition, audiological technicians assess the functioning of the balance systems (see page 109).

SPEECH THERAPIST

Speech and language therapists are highly trained specialists who play a major role in treating patients with voice and speech problems, and in the assessment and treatment of patients with swallowing difficulties (see page 131). Patients vary from children who need a little remedial help with speech production, to adults who have had the larynx removed and require extensive support to regain effective communication skills (see page 130). In such cases, the speech therapist helps to decide which method of re-establishing speech will be most appropriate, then guides the patient in ways of overcoming the various voice and speech-related difficulties experienced after surgery, until rehabilitation is as complete as is possible in the circumstances.

SPECIALIST SURGEONS

Many ENT surgeons are now specialising in narrower fields of expertise. These sub-specialties include:
• otology – ear surgery
• skull base surgery
• rhinology – surgery on the nose and sinuses
• laryngology – voice and airway surgery
• head and neck surgery
• paediatric otolaryngology – ENT treatment for children.
Specialist head and neck surgeons, who are fully trained in ENT, now usually manage the majority of cases of head and neck tumours.

FINDING OUT WHAT IS WRONG

Diagnosis is the first step towards treatment and recovery from a problem, and the ENT clinic offers a whole range of investigative procedures designed to find out exactly what is wrong and why. Technological advances and modern teaching enable the specialists to analyse and treat problems – from a simple ear infection to a tumour – quicker and more effectively than ever before.

Medical history and examination

Doctors need to know as much as possible about a patient's medical history and current problems to determine the right treatment. At the consultation, the patient can describe symptoms and talk over any concerns.

LOOKING AT SYMPTOMS

Symptoms of many different conditions can affect your ears, nose and throat, and your doctor will need to know all about your symptoms to reach an accurate diagnosis, so be sure to mention everything, even if you are not sure if it is relevant.

Ear pain and hearing problems

Otalgia, the medical term for earache, can occur on the external part of the ear, or deeper inside. However, earache does not necessarily indicate that the problem originates in the ear. Some of the nerves that supply the ear also supply other regions, such as the throat and sinuses, and a problem in these areas may cause 'referred' pain in the ears. A doctor who suspects that pain in an ear is referred will examine the mouth, nose and sinuses as well as the ear itself.

Swimming and ear infections
Swimming does not cause middle ear infections, although diving can be a contributory factor. A swim in polluted water, however, may cause an outer ear infection.

Deafness or hearing loss can occur suddenly or gradually, and can affect one or both ears. Hearing loss in children is a particular concern, as learning can suffer unless the cause is identified and treated promptly.

Tinnitus is the sensation of a ringing or buzzing noise in the ear that only the sufferer can hear. A precise description of the noise is important, as tinnitus may be a feature of several different conditions (see page 152).

Common causes of ear infections

The two basic types of ear infection are otitis externa, or outer ear infection, and otitis media, middle ear infection.

• **Otitis media** occurs when the eustachian tube becomes blocked. When this happens bacteria, which can normally drain freely back into the nose and throat to be harmlessly swallowed, become trapped in the mucus in the tube and start to multiply. If the tiny hair cells are damaged, by a cold virus for example, the mucus cannot get rid of the bacteria. The tube most often becomes blocked because of an infection, irritants such as cigarette smoke, or an allergy. Any of these may produce swelling and increase the amount of mucus produced in an attempt to get rid of the invaders. The same agents that block the eustachian tube also enlarge the glands at its opening, in effect closing its outlet. The mucus and saliva produced by teething babies can also cause the eustachian tube to function poorly. Increases in air pressure – in a plane, for example – can flatten the tube, effectively blocking it.

• **Otitis externa** is caused by bacteria entering the ear canal. This can happen to anyone who swims in polluted water, for example. People who pick at, or fiddle with, their ears also run the risk of introducing bacteria into the ear.

Other ear-related problems

Fluid leaking from the ear may indicate a range of conditions. Pus signifies an infection; blood indicates an injury; and clear fluid may represent leakage of cerebrospinal fluid. The vast majority of cases of cerebrospinal fluid leakage result from trauma and, if identified and treated quickly with antibiotics and bed rest, get better without the need for surgery.

Your symptoms and lifestyle

If you are referred by your GP to an ENT clinic, you will need to provide the specialists with as much information as possible. Making notes before your appointment on the following factors will make the consultation more useful.

• *Details of any past medical conditions: these help to put the current condition into context, and help in its assessment and diagnosis. For example, a patient who has diabetes is more likely to suffer with recurrent and severe ear infections.*

• *The drug or treatment history of the current condition: this can be crucial. Knowledge that a patient with bleeding from the nose is taking the anticoagulant drug warfarin, for example, is of immense importance.*

• *Your family medical history: this gives doctors an indication of any illnesses which run in the family.*

• *Your job and lifestyle. Whether you work in an office or out of doors can be important, as can whether you swim, fly or dive as a hobby. Be honest about whether you drink alcohol or smoke, and how much, as this can provide useful additional information.*

Health checks
A hearing test is part of your baby's developmental check at between six and nine months. The health visitor will shake a rattle while your baby is distracted to check the response to a sound stimulus.

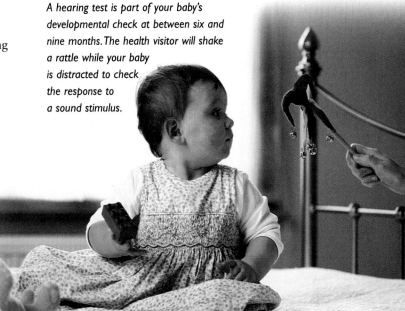

Dizziness is a vague term, so the doctor has to establish more precisely what kind of symptoms the patient is experiencing in order to diagnose the problem. Patients may feel that they or their surroundings are constantly moving or swirling around. This is known as vertigo, and is caused by a problem in the vestibular part of the inner ear. Less severe symptoms involving light-headedness, giddiness or disorientation are rarely due to problems originating in the inner ear. The duration of a dizzy feeling is important, too: dizziness lasting more than 24 hours may be caused by a viral infection of the vestibular system, while dizziness of much shorter duration is more likely to be due to Ménière's disease (see page 140).

A feeling of fullness in the ear is usually due to wax build-up, but it may indicate fluid in the middle ear.

The nose

A runny nose, sometimes accompanied by sneezing, usually indicates inflammation of the lining of the nose, or rhinitis. Patients with rhinitis may have a blocked nose, but this is more usual in those who have a deviated nasal septum, or obstruction such as nasal polyps or a tumour.

Bleeding from the nose – often an alarming symptom – usually stops easily with simple pressure and ice. Bleeding is rarely a cause for concern, but when it recurs and is from one nostril only, it may warrant investigation, as it may be a sign of a tumour.

Why are my ears so often blocked with wax?

Everybody's ears produce wax. In most cases, the small amounts made every day are naturally expelled from the ear, so the ears can be thought of as having their own 'self-cleaning' mechanism. However, there are many reasons why some people's ears seem to build up, rather than get rid of, wax. There may be an excessive amount of wax produced (often an inherited problem), or the ear canals may be unusually narrow, making the 'self-cleaning' process difficult. But by far the most common reason is the use of cottonwool buds to clean the ears: these can push more wax into the ears than they remove. Cotton buds can also damage the delicate skin of the ear canal. Common health wisdom states that you should never put anything in your ear that is smaller than your elbow.

ASK THE EXPERT

The sinuses

Facial pain occurring in between the eyes, on the side of the nose or in the forehead may be an indication of inflammation and obstruction of the sinuses. Patients who have a sinus infection may also complain of a poor sense of smell.

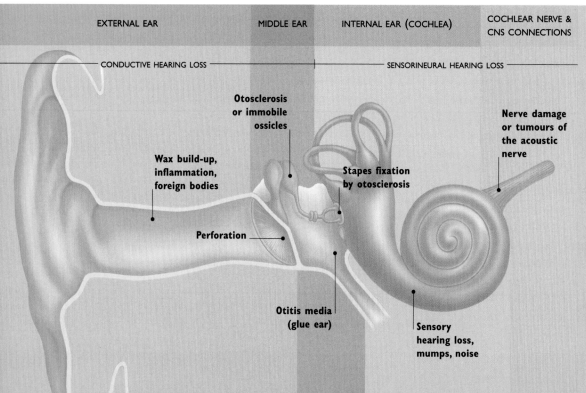

EXTERNAL EAR   MIDDLE EAR   INTERNAL EAR (COCHLEA)   COCHLEAR NERVE & CNS CONNECTIONS

CONDUCTIVE HEARING LOSS — SENSORINEURAL HEARING LOSS

Otosclerosis or immobile ossicles

Wax build-up, inflammation, foreign bodies

Nerve damage or tumours of the acoustic nerve

Stapes fixation by otosclerosis

Perforation

Otitis media (glue ear)

Sensory hearing loss, mumps, noise

Types of hearing loss

Hearing problems caused by injury to or blockage of the ear are termed conductive if they occur between the external ear and the stapes bone; those from the stapes into the inner ear are termed sensorineural. Different conditions cause problems in different areas.

The throat

Discomfort in the throat is usually a vague symptom, difficult to pinpoint to one specific area. It is most often due to infection, either in the lining of the throat (pharyngitis) or tonsils (tonsillitis). A lump in the throat is common and rarely points to serious underlying disease. It is often stress-related, but anyone who has difficulty in swallowing, or earache as well, needs further investigation.

The airway

Hoarseness is not unusual in patients who have a cold, or in people who overuse their voice on a regular basis, such as singers or teachers. Overuse of the voice can trigger the growth of nodules or polyps on the vocal cords within the larynx (voice box); these benign growths generally make the voice sound hoarse. Occasionally, the cause of a hoarse voice turns out to be a tumour on the cords.

Stridor is the term used to describe a harsh sound produced typically on breathing in, but it can also occur on breathing out. It indicates narrowing of the larynx or trachea, possibly caused by a partial obstruction.

EXAMINING THE EAR

Doctors begin an ear examination with a close look at the outer, visible part of the ear (the pinna), where a number of problems can be identified. Some injuries can result in a blood clot beneath the skin of the ear. This is known as haematoma auris. An abscess may develop either in a previously formed blood clot or on its own. A blood clot or abscess can destroy the cartilage of the outer ear, and if this is left untreated it may eventually lead to scarring, resulting in 'cauliflower ear'. Treatment involves the removal of the clot and drainage of the abscess.

Basal and squamous cell cancers – tumours related to sun exposure – are also common on the external ear, but can be effectively treated using photodynamic therapy.

Using an otoscope

External examination is followed by inspection of the ear canal and eardrum with an otoscope. This provides the doctor with a view of the ear canal, and of the middle ear, through the semi-transparent eardrum. If earwax blocks the view, the doctor removes the wax first. The otoscope enables the doctor to diagnose a range of ear problems such as eczema of the ear canal, which can become infected, particularly if the ear is not dried after a swim or shower. It is also possible to see boils or abscesses.

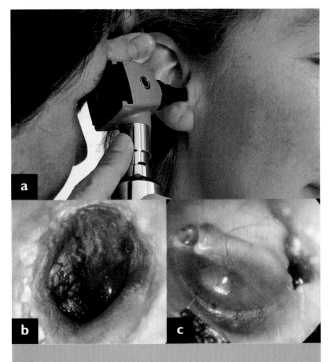

The view through an otoscope

a To examine the ear using an otoscope, the doctor gently pulls on the outer ear in order to straighten the ear canal to get a better view along it. The instrument is not inserted deeply: the light on its end enables the doctor to see to the eardrum and beyond.

b In a case of otitis media, a doctor would see redness and bulging of the eardrum, caused by fluid build-up behind it.

c In persistent cases of otitis media the eardrum may appear dull, and there might be fewer blood vessels than normal on its surface.

The appearance of the eardrum may give a clue as to the state of health of the middle ear. For example, fluid in the middle ear may cause bulging of the eardrum, and alter its surface colour and degree of transparency. Perforations or infections may also affect the eardrum. Through the eardrum it is also possible to see the ossicles. In patients who have had previous surgery or recurrent chronic infections the ossicles may have eroded or be missing altogether, which can be a cause of hearing loss.

Using a microscope

For a more detailed look at the middle ear, the doctor will use a microscope, which magnifies the ear canal and eardrum. The use of a microscope also enables simple procedures to be carried out in the ENT clinic, including the removal of excessive wax or foreign bodies.

Examining the eustachian tubes

It is difficult for doctors to determine how well the eustachian tubes are working by otoscopic examination, but they can get an indication by checking the appearance of the eardrums. Patients with poor eustachian tube function are unable to force air into the tubes by simply pinching the nose and breathing out. This creates within the middle ear a negative pressure that can 'suck in' the eardrum, drawing it away from the canal, and this can be seen with an otoscope. It does not prove that there is a problem with the eustachian tubes, however, so further examination is necessary.

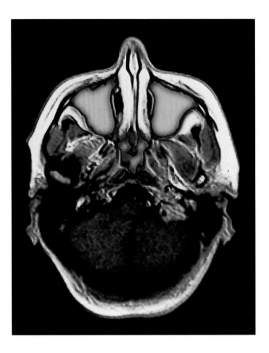

Inside the human head
This false-colour image produced from an MRI scan of a cross-section through the head shows the nose at top centre, the maxillary sinuses in yellow and the sphenoidal sinuses in orange.

Ear examination is usually supplemented by tests of hearing and balance (see pages 107–9).

EXAMINING THE NOSE AND SINUSES

An examination of the nose starts with the doctor looking at its external appearance and shape. If there is a deformity, was it present at birth or due to an injury? The specialist must make this distinction because trauma-related deformities may be associated with injuries in other parts of the face not otherwise immediately apparent, such as fractures of the lower rim of the eye socket or damage to the teeth. Doctors also take a look at the overall symmetry of the face. Swelling and/or tenderness could indicate possible sinus infection.

Looking inside the nose

To start with, a doctor uses a speculum to hold the nostrils open and shines a light inside to look at the front of the nasal cavity. The back of the nose can be viewed using an angled mirror placed inside the mouth. The central part of the nose, however, can only be properly inspected with a fibreoptic telescope – flexible or rigid. A flexible telescope is generally used for examining the throat, larynx and back of the nose. Rigid telescopes are used mainly to examine the nose and the sinuses.

Some patients who have had sinus surgery have large, open sinus cavities that are easily visible. In general, however, a doctor can't get a complete view of normal sinuses by examining the nose with a nasal speculum or an angled rigid telescope. Instead, the patient is sent to a clinic for further investigations, such as imaging tests.

EXAMINING THE THROAT

This investigation begins with a look at the patient's neck, which is best examined by palpation (gentle feeling) of the main structures. The key structures that concern an ENT

EXPERIENCING A TELESCOPE NASAL EXAMINATION

I had been feeling as if my nose was blocked on and off for some months. My GP referred me to an ENT clinic where the doctor examined my nose using a telescope.

Before the telescope was inserted, the doctor sprayed my nostrils with a decongestant and anaesthetic, which he told me was derived from cocaine. Over a period of about five minutes this relaxed my nostrils (which I wasn't really conscious of). He then started to insert the rigid telescope.

I was conscious of the instrument being in my nose but there was no pain or even discomfort. The doctor passed the telescope up into one nostril and manoeuvred it into my nasal cavity. He then removed it and inserted it in my other nostril. He told me that he had found a polyp in my left nostril and put me on the waiting list to have it removed. The whole examination took only 15 minutes, including the wait for the anaesthetic to take effect.

HAVING AN INDIRECT LARYNGOSCOPY

My doctor was unable to tell why my voice was so hoarse when I didn't have a sore throat or a cold, so referred me to the local ENT clinic for a specialist examination of my larynx and vocal cords by indirect laryngoscopy.

The specialist at the clinic explained that he was going to position a special angled mirror within my mouth to obtain as good a view as possible of my larynx and vocal cords. Just before the examination began, he heated the mirror very slightly so that it wouldn't steam up when I breathed

on it. He asked me to concentrate on breathing through my mouth as normally as possible all through the examination.

I was asked to open my mouth and stick out my tongue, which the doctor gently grasped and pulled forward with a gauze swab. He then introduced the mirror into my mouth and positioned it so that it was touching the soft palate on the roof of my mouth, just in front of the uvula. Luckily I was able to stay relaxed and not gag. The doctor asked me to say a prolonged 'e' so that my epiglottis would rise and he could see

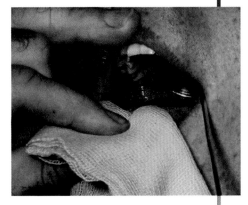

into my larynx. Before I began to feel too uncomfortable, the doctor withdrew the mirror, explaining that he would replace it after I'd had a short rest. After several short examinations, the doctor said the test was over.

specialist are the lymph glands, which can easily be felt where they sit on either side of the Adam's apple, close to the major blood vessels. Lymph glands may be affected by tumours that originate in the mucosal lining of the throat, the base of the tongue, the nasopharynx (back of the nose) or the larynx.

Other structures in the neck that can require assessment include the thyroid gland. As this is in the lower part of the neck, it is not easy to feel in most people. If the specialist can easily feel the thyroid gland, it is probably enlarged, due to an autoimmune disorder such as Graves disease, or to a tumour, which needs further investigation.

Looking inside the mouth

The oral cavity – the tongue, tonsils, back wall of the throat and lining of the mouth – is easily examined using a good headlight and two strong tongue depressors. The parotid salivary gland, in front of the ear, drains saliva into the mouth opposite the upper second molar tooth, and this point in the mouth is demarcated by a prominent hillock which is easy to see. In addition, the floor of the mouth contains the salivary glands that drain saliva into the mouth. There may be cysts or swellings in these areas.

Examining the larynx is more difficult. It can be done in the ENT clinic either with a flexible telescope, or by a technique known as 'indirect laryngoscopy'.

Indirect laryngoscopy

During an indirect laryngoscopy, the doctor introduces an angled mirror on the end of a long metal stalk into the mouth and uses it to examine the epiglottis, tongue base and interior of the larynx, and – when necessary – the upper part of the trachea. The vocal cords can be seen and their movement assessed – if a vocal cord is paralysed, it will not move when the patient talks or sings, as requested by the doctor.

One problem with indirect laryngoscopy is that some patients have a strong gag reflex and cannot tolerate a mirror pushed towards their throat. Local anaesthetic spray can sometimes suppress this reflex so that the doctor can proceed with the examination. If this does not work, however, a specialist must use a flexible fibreoptic nasoendoscope, which is passed up one of the nostrils and through the nasal passages behind (see page 111).

Direct laryngoscopy

Sometimes the doctor wants to examine the internal structures of the larynx in more detail, perhaps to take biopsies of abnormal-looking tissue. This is done with the patient under a general anaesthetic in the operating theatre, where the specialist has access to a range of rigid endoscopes. This examination of the larynx is known as direct (as opposed to indirect) laryngoscopy.

Videostroboscopy

This is the latest way of viewing and recording the vocal cords. A stroboscope is fed down the throat and into the larynx, where the cords are filmed in action, in a process called videostroboscopy.

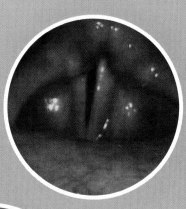

Tighter
The vocal cords narrow as the patient sounds a sustained vowel.

What is it used for?

The movements of the vocal cords are complex and the focus of much research. The creation of sound is no longer thought to be a simple case of the two vocal cords moving in and out against each other during speech. Each vocal cord is covered by a thin sheet of highly specialised mucosa that moves in a fluid manner by means of a series of rapid oscillations. This oscillatory movement is at a rate faster than the eye can detect: the only way to view the mucosal wave is via a videostroboscopy. This allows earlier detection than was previously possible of growths, scarring, broken blood vessels, and all manner of abnormalities and malfunctioning.

How does it work?

The examination involves the use of a stroboscope – a flexible telescope with a tiny camera and strobe light. Light is directed down the scope at a rate that effectively 'freeze-frames' the moving mucosal wave at a slightly different phase each time. The wave is seen to advance slowly, step by step, and any abnormalities in the construction of the wave can be more easily detected. The camera records the images and projects them, frame by frame, onto a TV monitor. Filming is in real time, but the specialist will later play back sequences in slow motion, or examine images as a series of still photos. The patient is awake throughout and is usually asked to vocalise various sounds so the vocal cords can be filmed in action.

VIDEOSTROBOSCOPY IN ACTION

The vocal cords viewed through a stroboscope, as they appear on a television monitor. The cords are two bands of muscle, flanked by the ventricular folds.

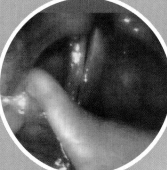

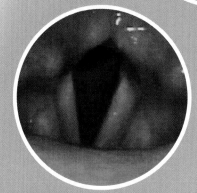

Taut
The vocal cords are pulled taut as the patient intones a prolonged 'eeee' followed by a prolonged 'aaah'.

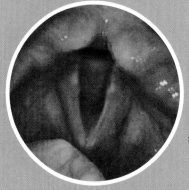

Breathing out
As the patient breathes out the vocal cords relax and open to allow air to be exhaled from the lungs.

Breathing in
The cords also open when the patient breathes in, so air can pass down the larynx, into the trachea and to the lungs.

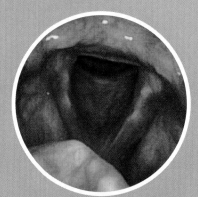

Taking a deep breath
The vocal cords are wide open as the patient takes a deep breath.

Hearing tests

The many different hearing tests available at an ENT clinic range from simple whispering to the use of a computerised probe. They are designed to assess whether a patient's hearing is impaired, and if so to what degree and what is causing the problem.

WHISPER TESTS

A specialist can gain a rough idea as to the level of hearing by conducting some simple 'whisper' tests, whereby a number or a short word is whispered into each ear at varying distances. This is only a crude test and will need verification by a formal hearing assessment.

TUNING FORK TESTS

The Rinne and Weber tests, performed in sequence, assess the type and extent of hearing loss. They use a standard tuning fork with a resonant frequency of 512Hz. A higher resonance might not be heard easily; anything lower might be felt as well as heard, confusing the test's result.

How do they work?

- **The Rinne test** is aimed at finding out how well a patient hears a sound transmitted to the middle and inner ear by air conduction (AC), in comparison with the same sound transmitted by bone conduction (BC) through vibration of the bony skull that vibrates the inner ear.
- **The Weber test** will detect whether a tuning fork placed at a midpoint between the ears is heard predominantly in just one ear.

What can they tell us?

Patients whose hearing is within the normal range hear AC better than BC, and detect the tuning fork in the Weber test equally well with both ears.

Patients whose hearing loss is due to a problem with the conductive mechanisms of the middle ear should hear BC better than AC, because of a reduction in sound transmission by AC. These patients will hear the tuning fork in the Weber test more clearly in the ear with the conductive abnormality.

Patients whose hearing loss is caused by a problem with the neural connections to the brain – where the mechanisms transmitting sound to the inner ear are intact – will hear AC better than BC, since both will be reduced in proportion to each other. But the tuning fork in the Weber test will be heard best in the better hearing ear, rather than the ear where hearing is more impaired.

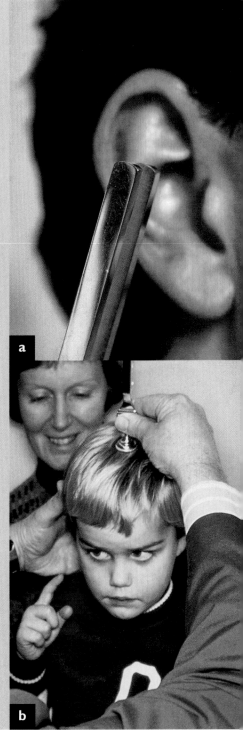

Rinne test

a A tuning fork is struck and then placed next to one ear. If the patient hears the sound, it is being transmitted by air conduction (AC). While the tuning fork is still resonating, its base is placed against the mastoid process (the bony protrusion behind the ear). If the patient hears the sound this time, it is being transmitted by bone conduction (BC). The process is repeated for the other ear.

Weber test

b The tuning fork is struck and then placed either in the middle of the forehead or on the vertex (highest point) of the head, in line with the centre of the nose. The specialist records whether the patient hears the sound, and if so whether it is heard equally in both ears, or mainly in one ear or the other.

AUDIOMETRY

An audiometry test is carried out at an ENT clinic in a soundproof room. The test is designed to measure air conduction (AC) and bone conduction (BC) thresholds.

How does it work?

To test for AC thresholds, the patient wears headphones so that the only sound which can be heard is that produced by the audiometer – the hearing test machine. Common practice is to test hearing at distinct set frequencies only, usually 250Hz, 500Hz, 1kHz, 2kHz, 4kHz and 8kHz. At each frequency, a sound is played to each ear in turn, and the patient must press a button to indicate that he or she heard the sound. The loudness or intensity of the sound is gradually decreased until the patient does not respond. The quietest sound at which the patient registers a response is termed the threshold for that particular frequency. This is repeated for the remaining frequencies, and then for the other ear.

The technician makes up a graph to show the hearing thresholds for each frequency. The level, or loudness, of sound is measured in decibels, or dB. This is a logarithmic scale, which means that a sound measured at 20dB has in fact ten times the sound intensity of a sound of 10dB, not twice the intensity.

The audiological technician can test BC thresholds by applying a special bone vibrator to the mastoid process (the prominent bony protrusion behind the ear), then following the same procedure. With both AC and BC tests completed, the specialist can then examine any differences in the AC and BC thresholds.

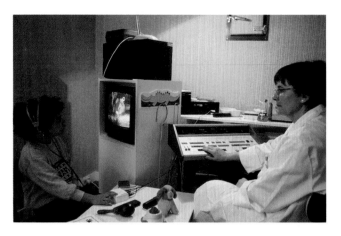

Audiometric hearing test
The audiological technician sends sounds of varying volume through the earphones worn by the child, and the child presses a button whenever a sound is heard. To make the test more interesting, the sounds are associated with pictures on a television monitor.

TYMPANOMETRY

This hearing test helps the ENT specialist to assess the functioning of the eustachian tubes, and – if there is an abnormality – whether treatment is necessary, or possible.

How does it work?

The audiologist inserts a probe into the outer part of the patient's ear canal. The probe calculates the eardrum's movement at different pressures produced by the probe, and thereby gains an impression of the pressure within the middle ear. Maximum movement of the drum occurs when pressure produced by the probe in the canal is equal to pressure within the middle ear. A computer attached to the probe produces a graph to show the test results.

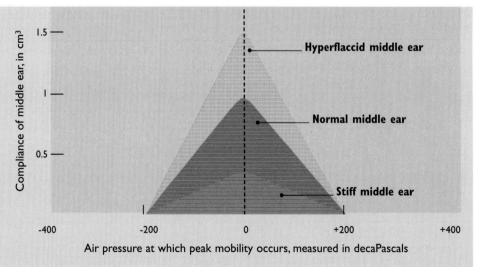

Tympanogram

The test measures the level of mobility (compliance) of ossicles within the middle ear with varying air pressures. Low mobility shows the eardrum and ossicles are stiff or obstructed; the likely cause is fluid in the middle ear. High mobility shows the drum is too flaccid, and may indicate damage.

Compliance of middle ear, in cm³

1.5 —

1 —

0.5 —

Hyperflaccid middle ear

Normal middle ear

Stiff middle ear

-400   -200   0   +200   +400

Air pressure at which peak mobility occurs, measured in decaPascals

Tests of balance

In addition to testing hearing, audiology departments also perform balance tests. ENT specialists may request one of these tests for a patient who is suffering from vertigo (severe dizziness) for which there is no obvious cause.

There are various balance tests, each one designed to assess a separate aspect of the balance mechanism. If results are to be accurate, it is vital that patients stop taking any sedatives designed to suppress disturbances of the inner ear at least 48 hours before a test takes place.

NYSTAGMUS: THE KEY TO BALANCE TESTING

If a patient experiences the dizziness known as vertigo, it is often due to an abnormality in the inner ear balance system within one ear or the other. The brain receives incorrect information from the abnormal side to indicate that the body is spinning in one particular direction, and therefore compensates by causing the eyes to undergo rapid, involuntary oscillatory movements towards the opposite side. These eye movements are called nystagmus.

ENT experts categorise nystagmus according to its direction (mainly to the left or right) or its degree, which is related to the severity of the inner ear abnormality. These parameters can be recorded by a technique known as electronystagmography (ENG), in which an audiological technician attaches electrodes to the skin close to the patient's eyes; the electrodes detect minute changes in the electrical potential generated by even the tiniest of eye movements.

CALORIC TESTS

Caloric testing is done to determine whether the patient has a diseased labyrinth. (This is the fluid-filled system of coiled bony tubes that makes up the inner ear and, among other things, controls balance.) Some people feel uncomfortable or even dizzy when cold or warm water is squirted into their ear. It is this phenomenon which forms the basis of the tests, in which water of two different temperatures – 30°C and 44°C – is introduced into each ear in turn.

The resulting change of temperature within the inner ear triggers motion currents in the fluid contained within the labyrinth. This may give rise to a sensation of dizziness in the patient, followed by nystagmus. The degree of the nystagmus (measured by ENG) varies according to the severity of the patient's condition; the

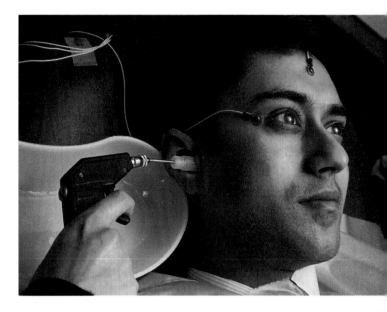

Caloric test in action
The electrodes attached to the patient's skin, above and beside his eyes, measure involuntary eye movement by electronystagmography (ENG). This indicates what degree of dizziness, if any, is being induced by the water being squirted into his ear.

direction varies according to the temperature of the water. If the labyrinth is healthy, nystagmus will occur for a predictable period. If there is a problem, nystagmus will occur for a short time, or not at all.

ROTATORY CHAIR TEST

This test stimulates nystagmus, so that it can be measured accurately. A patient with a diseased inner ear becomes less dizzy than a person with healthy ears. The patient sits, with eyes closed, in a swivel-type chair. The audiologist then spins the chair around ten times in a total time of 20 seconds, then brings the chair to an abrupt stop. This procedure will cause nystagmus in almost all patients, and the audiologist records the direction and degree manually or via ENG.

Care must be taken when performing a rotatory chair test, particularly with patients suffering from severe vertigo, as the stimulus is fairly significant and can make the condition worse.

Investigative tests of the nose

When doctors test the working of the nose, they are looking to establish the cause of a variety of problems and abnormalities. Tests fall into three main categories: allergy tests, tests to assess a patient's sense of smell, and tests on the behaviour of the nasal hairs.

ALLERGY TESTS

As such a large number of patients suffer from allergic rhinitis, it is hardly surprising that allergy tests are among the most common investigations to take place in the ENT clinic. They usually involve provoking then observing a series of skin reactions to a variety of different allergens (substances that can provoke an allergic reaction), including grass pollen, house dust, house-dust mites, cat and dog hairs, feathers and milk. The ENT nurse places a small quantity of protein prepared from each allergen onto a patient's forearm. If the patient is allergic to any of the substances, a reddish, slightly raised weal will appear.

The tests may not be valid if the patient is taking antihistamine tablets, such as for hay fever, as these will reduce any allergic response to the test substances. In such circumstances, the clinic nurse and doctor will probably decide to postpone the test until the patient has been free from the drug for a period of at least 48 hours.

TESTS ASSESSING THE SENSE OF SMELL

Olfactory tests – tests of the sense of smell – aim to evaluate the range of smells a patient can pick up, and how well the odours are detected. The simplest olfactory test involves presenting a range of standard liquid odours to the patient, which the patient is asked to identify. This is a crude test, because results are dependent on the patient already being familiar with all the smells on offer.

More accurate is electro-olfactography (EOG), in which an electrode is placed alongside the olfactory nasal lining, high in the nasal cavity. The patient sniffs a succession of odours, and the electrode detects the electrical potential generated by the olfactory cells in response to each odour.

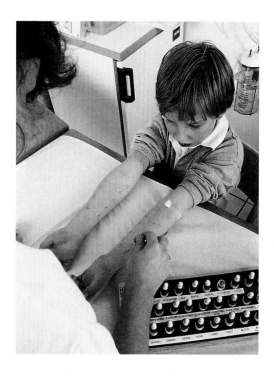

Testing for a reaction
This boy's arms are being painted with a variety of allergens to try to pinpoint which is causing his allergic rhinitis.

MUCOCILIARY FUNCTION TESTING

The nasal lining is covered by a layer of highly specialised cilia (tiny hair-like structures) that beat at a rate of approximately 15 times per second to move overlying mucus to the back of the nose so it can be swallowed. This is known as mucociliary clearance or transport. It can be measured by placing a drop of saccharin just inside the nose and asking the patient to swallow every 30 seconds. The time taken for the patient to experience a sweet taste should be 12 to 15 minutes if ciliary beat frequency is normal. If it takes longer than this, there is a problem with ciliary function.

Alzheimer's disease and the sense of smell

TALKING POINT

Many specialists now think that the inability to recognise once-familiar smells – combined with a lack of awareness that the sense of smell is deteriorating – can be an early indicator of Alzheimer's disease. Alzheimer's is a type of dementia in which degeneration of brain tissue leads to increasing loss of memory and progressively disorganised reasoning and behaviour. But doctors stress that a deterioration in the sense of smell is not by any means a certain indicator of the disease and should not be interpreted as such.

Looking inside the nose and throat

Of all the methods used by ENT specialists to examine the interior of the nose, the pharynx and larynx, flexible nasopharyngoscopy is probably the most effective.

A nasopharyngoscopy is a test in which a doctor – generally an ENT specialist – uses a flexible fibreoptic nasoendoscope to examine a patient's upper airway. The doctor may be looking for problems or abnormalities in the nose, but the procedure is most commonly employed to make a detailed examination of the throat and larynx.

Fibreoptic cabling within the nasoendoscope's narrow tubing transmits images from within the patient's head and neck to the eye of the specialist via an optical system or a miniature video camera. If a video camera is used, the examination can be displayed on a monitor there and then, or recorded and played back later, or both.

The specialist usually guides the tip of the nasoendoscope down the throat via the patient's nose. This is because introducing it through the mouth can trigger the gag reflex, which might make the patient jerk their head or even bite on the end of the scope.

A long and winding road
The doctor looks down the eye piece of the nasoendoscope as he guides the instrument's tubing up through one of the patient's nostrils, along the nasal passages and down the throat.

EXPERIENCING A FLEXIBLE NASOPHARYNGOSCOPY

My doctor thought a closer look at my throat and larynx was needed and so referred me to the ENT clinic for an examination with a flexible nasoendoscope.

The doctor sprayed one of my nostrils with a combined anaesthetic and decongestant that took about three minutes to take effect. With the nostril quite numb, he gently guided the scope up my nose, while looking through the eye piece. When he was sure the scope had reached the back of my nose, he used the controls to angle it in a downward direction. The doctor guided it past the soft palate, the back wall of the pharynx and the base of my tongue, so that he could see any abnormalities. Finally, it reached my larynx, at which point he asked me to sing the letter 'e', so that he could assess the movements of my vocal cords.

Once the doctor was happy that he had seen all there was to see, he carefully removed the scope. Much to my relief, it hadn't turned out to be a painful process, although I had felt a bit uncomfortable.

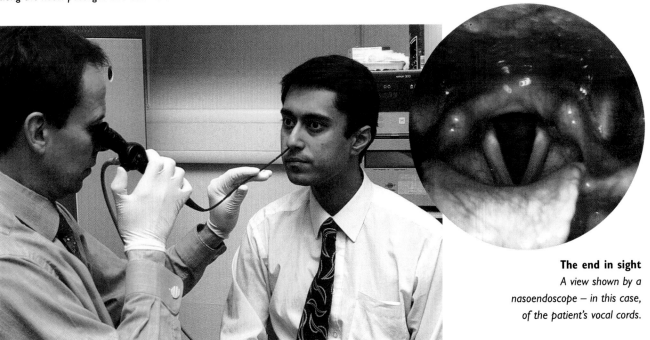

The end in sight
A view shown by a nasoendoscope – in this case, of the patient's vocal cords.

Investigating a lump in the neck

Swellings or lumps in the neck often cause patients great concern. In order to allay their fears, GPs fast-track a significant proportion to the ENT clinic for speedy diagnosis. The good news is that in most cases the swellings are benign.

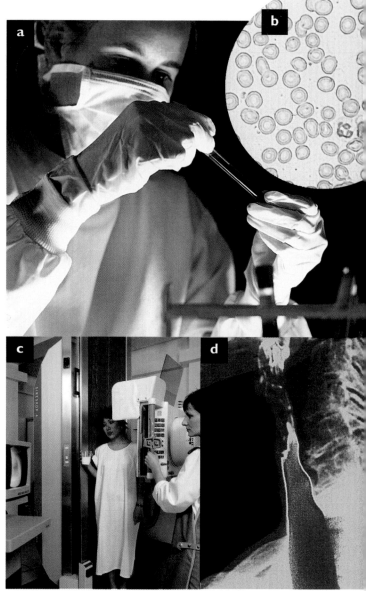

CAUSES FOR CONCERN

Features in the patient's history which may be cause for concern include a sudden, rapid enlargement in a swelling in the neck, and the presence of deep, unrelenting pain which does not respond to simple painkillers. A breakdown in the skin overlying a lesion, or symptoms from within the pharynx or other internal structures – such as a lump, difficulty swallowing, hoarseness of the voice or earache due to referred pain – are also symptoms the doctor will want to investigate.

INITIAL INVESTIGATIONS

The specialist will carry out a thorough examination of the neck, look into the mouth, nose and ears, and then perform a flexible nasoendoscopy in order to study all aspects of the pharynx and larynx. The investigative process continues with blood tests to establish the state of the patient's blood before treatment begins, including whether the patient is anaemic, what chemicals are dissolved in the plasma and whether there are any traces of infection in the blood.

A chest X-ray follows, to check whether there is an associated lung tumour. The X-ray is also used to check for any signs of a chest infection or potential heart failure, which may put the patient at risk if a general anaesthetic becomes necessary at some future date.

In addition to these tests, the specialist selects the tests which are the most appropriate for each individual case.

BARIUM SWALLOW, OR VIDEOFLUOROSCOPY

The specialist may recommend a barium swallow, particularly if a key symptom is difficulty in swallowing. In this procedure, the patient swallows a radio-opaque barium-containing liquid which lines the pharynx and oesophagus, and shows up brightly when the radiologist takes X-ray pictures. This test highlights any lesion that is narrowing the pharynx or oesophagus, which may have been out of view of the nasoendoscopic examination.

ASPIRATING A LUMP

Fine-needle aspiration cytology (FNAC) has revolutionised the assessment of patients with cancerous and benign neck swellings by allowing doctors to obtain samples of tissue without the patient having to undergo surgery. It is also used as an aid in the diagnosis of lumps in other parts of the body, including the breast. The test is carried out by an ENT specialist or by a cytopathologist (a specialist in the study of cells). A needle and syringe is used to draw out a sample of material from the lump. The needle is fine enough to avoid aspirating blood as well as cells. The material from the lump is sent to the laboratory for analysis at once, and the results of the test are often available just a few hours later.

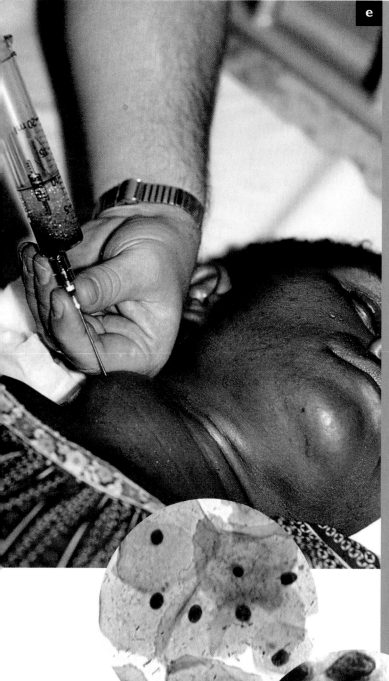

Three common diagnostic tests

a and **b** Taking a blood sample

A technician examines a blood sample in a test tube. Shown inset are highly magnified blood cells taken from a patient with anaemia. Because the red blood cells lack iron, an essential component of the blood pigment haemoglobin, they stain poorly. (Just two white blood cells are identifiable, both stained purple.). Anaemia is a symptom, not a disease, so a specialist must now identify the disorder that is causing the anaemia. There is a possibility that it could be cancer.

c and **d** A barium swallow

A patient stands ready to take a swallow from a glass of barium meal and follow its progress on the monitor attached to the digital X-ray system. The drink contains barium sulphate, a substance opaque to X-rays that outlines regions of the digestive tract. Here, the pharynx and oesophagus are being checked for abnormalities such as a tumour. The coloured X-ray shows as red the oesophagus of a patient who is in the act of swallowing barium meal – the upper part of the oesophagus appears narrow as muscles constrict to swallow the drink.

e Having a lump aspirated

The patient is undergoing a fine-needle aspiration cytology (FNAC) test as part of an investigation into a lump in her thyroid gland. The aim of the test is to remove a small quantity of cells from within the lump, and send them to the laboratory for immediate analysis. A local anaesthetic can cause more discomfort afterwards than the procedure itself, so the patient is not anaesthetised. After cleaning the skin with a swab, the specialist inserts a needle attached to a syringe into the lump and, making several 'passes', draws out the tissue needed, which is then smeared onto several glass slides and sent to the laboratory.

Normal and cancerous cells

These two cell samples – seen here stained and magnified – were removed by FNAC from tissue from two different patients. They demonstrate the striking difference between normal squamous cells (far right) and cancerous squamous cells (near right).

Cancers of the head and neck that are diagnosed while still small and localised have a cure rate of over 80 per cent.

Microbiological testing

Many patients arrive at ENT clinics with an infection, such as an inflamed, painful ear or acute tonsillitis. Microbiological testing enables the consultant to identify the organism responsible for the infection – the pathogen – so that the most effective drugs can be prescribed.

TAKING A SAMPLE

The first stage is to take a sample of the infected area and send it to the laboratory for analysis. In the case of an infection of the external part of the ear canal, for example, it is easy enough to take a swab of the inflammatory discharge in the ear canal.

If the patient has an infection of the middle ear, the eardrum may be bulging, red and inflamed, indicating that there is infected fluid, known as an effusion, in the middle ear. The pain can sometimes be so severe that it has to be relieved by making a tiny incision in the eardrum to release the fluid; when this happens, some of the fluid can be sent for analysis.

In the case of a neck abscess, a sample of the contents can be drawn out using a needle and syringe.

CULTURING THE SAMPLE

Once the sample has reached the laboratory, a microbiology technician distributes it evenly across the surface of a specialised agar jelly plate. The plate is then incubated in a warm environment for 48 hours. At the end of this period, the pathogens (the micro-organisms causing the infection) in the sample will have multiplied, making analysis easier. In the case of hardier organisms an incubation period of up to six weeks is often necessary.

IDENTIFYING THE PATHOGEN

The microbiologist removes part of the colony of organisms and places it on a glass slide for examination under a microscope. Each organism has a unique appearance, enabling the microbiologist to make a precise identification. Viruses are so small that they cannot be examined using an ordinary light microscope, however.

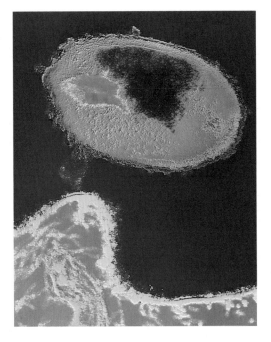

Diphtheria bacterium
A rod-shaped diphtheria bacterium (shown here in cross-section) lies on the surface of the throat. Treatment is with antitoxins and penicillin.

Instead, the microbiologist must use an electron microscope, which provides magnification a thousand times greater than a light microscope.

TAKING A FULL BLOOD COUNT

A full blood count (FBC) can help to establish the seriousness of the infection, by telling the specialist the total white blood cell count of the patient. In the presence of an infection, the number of white cells will usually have increased. If a patient has leukaemia, however, the number of white cells may actually have fallen, rather than increased, making it difficult for the patient to resist even the mildest of infections.

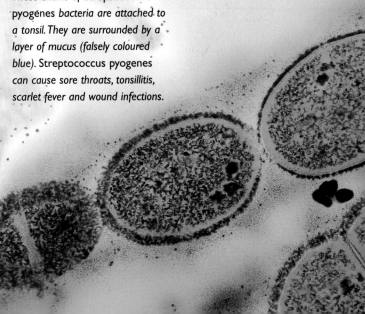

Streptococcus bacteria
These chains of Streptococcus pyogenes bacteria are attached to a tonsil. They are surrounded by a layer of mucus (falsely coloured blue). Streptococcus pyogenes can cause sore throats, tonsillitis, scarlet fever and wound infections.

Imaging techniques

The tools that enable doctors to visualise the structures within the body that can't otherwise be seen – notably X-ray and scanning machines – are invaluable in the ENT clinic. These tools can locate tumours, establish the severity of conditions such as sinusitis and even find foreign objects such as fish bones.

X-RAYS

In spite of newer developments in imaging techniques, X-rays are still a vital detecting tool for diseases and disorders of the ears, nose and throat. For example, if a patient has accidentally swallowed a fish bone that may have lodged itself somewhere in the pharynx, an X-ray can help the specialist to identify where the bone is. For patients with acute sinusitis, an X-ray of the sinuses will often help to diagnose the severity of the condition. However, a patient with a fractured nose does not usually require an X-ray, since a doctor can diagnose a fractured nose by physical examination.

CT SCANNING

Computerised tomography (CT) scanning is particularly useful in ENT because many of the structures of the ears, nose and throat can't be seen properly even with the aid of telescopes and nasoendoscopy. During a CT scan, a series of X-rays are directed at the specific area in question, from a variety of angles and planes. The points at which the X-ray beams intersect enable the scanner's computer to calculate precisely how much of the X-ray beam has been absorbed by the tissue. In this way, the computer produces a detailed picture of the target area, highlighting both normal structures and abnormal lesions.

CT scanning is used for examining the sinuses in more detail than an X-ray can provide, mapping out the lymph glands in the neck in cases of suspected cancer, and visualising the middle ear and mastoid system for evidence of chronic infections.

MRI

Magnetic resonance imaging (MRI) employs magnets rather than X-rays to scan the body. The patient is asked to lie on a couch, which then slowly moves through what is in effect a long, hollow, cylindrical magnet. The magnet causes a realignment of the hydrogen atoms present within the cells of the area under investigation. When the hydrogen atoms assume their original state, there is a loss of energy. The MRI computer detects this

Images of the head

a A computerised tomography (CT) scan presents a profile of a human head, with bone shown as pink or blue, and soft tissue – including the nasal cavity and throat – coloured yellow or green.

b Magnetic resonance imaging (MRI) techniques produced these cross-sections through a human head, facing forward. The coloured image clearly shows the nasal cavity, flanked on either side by the air-filled maxillary sinuses.

shift in energy and converts it into an electronic form. The sum total of all of the energy shifts is then compiled into a detailed image.

MRI is mainly used in the ENT clinic to diagnose small tumours of the auditory nerve, swellings related to the salivary glands, and (occasionally) tumours of the sinuses.

Whereas CT scanning is especially good at imaging bony structures, MRI scanning's strength lies in detecting soft tissues including muscle, glands and fat. The advantage of MRI is that the patient avoids exposure to X-rays, but many patients find MRI claustrophobic. Also, metallic implants in the body, such as artificial hips, heart valves or pacemakers can interfere with the magnetic image, and the magnetic field can also interfere with the implants themselves. The radiologist makes the final decision as to whether it is safe to proceed with the scan.

CURRENT TREATMENTS

Many ear, nose and throat problems can be resolved with the help of drugs; others need treatment in the form of surgery. Some surgical procedures are minor and can be performed in the outpatients department under local anaesthetic, whereas others – notably operations to restore hearing – require a spell in hospital followed by rehabilitation. Whatever the patient's condition and treatment, staff at the ENT clinic are there to help, using cutting-edge diagnostic and surgical equipment, coupled with specialist expertise.

Drug therapy

Today's advanced drugs are designed to target and treat a whole range of ear, nose and throat conditions, from severe vertigo to the common cold.

Drugs can be administered either topically or systemically. Topical drugs are applied to the surface to be treated, for example the skin or nasal lining, and take the form of cream or ointment, drops or spray. They deliver the drug to the targeted area and minimise its absorption into the bloodstream. Systemic drugs are swallowed or injected, after which they are absorbed into the bloodstream, which distributes them to the targeted areas of the body.

DRUGS FOR EAR CONDITIONS

Drugs for the external parts of the ear are usually given topically, generally in the form of drops. In cases of severe ear infection, discharge in the ear canal will need to be cleared by microsuction. If the ear canal is very swollen, the doctor will insert a small foam wick that soaks up the drops and allows them to reach the infected ear canal. The wick is left in place for a few days.

- **Drops for hardened wax in the ear** Wax can be softened by adding warm olive oil to the ear canal, or a solution of sodium bicarbonate and water, or one of the many proprietary eardrops available over the counter. One of these may be sufficient by itself to clear the wax; if not, the doctor can remove it by syringing or microsuction.

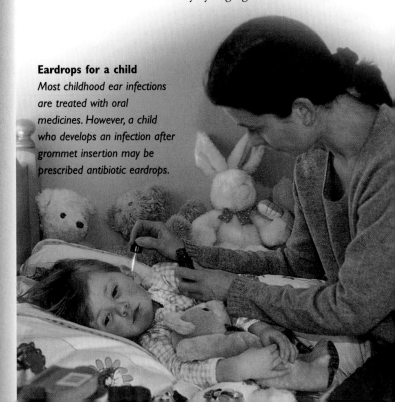

Eardrops for a child
Most childhood ear infections are treated with oral medicines. However, a child who develops an infection after grommet insertion may be prescribed antibiotic eardrops.

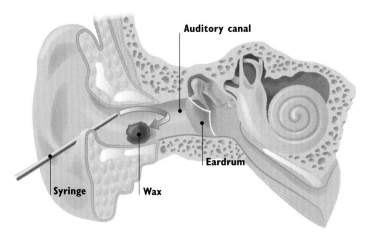

Auditory canal

Eardrum

Syringe **Wax**

Syringing an ear
The syringe squirts water upward so that it falls behind the blockage and forces the wax out of the ear. This must be performed by trained personnel using the correct equipment to avoid damage to the ear.

- **Antibiotic eardrops for the outer ear** An external ear inflammation (otitis externa) due to bacterial infection is generally safely and effectively treated with antibiotic eardrops. Occasionally, the drops cause an allergic skin reaction. A combination of antibiotic and steroid (in drop form) will reduce this reaction, and help to reduce swelling of the skin in the infected ear canal.
- **Antibiotics for the middle ear** Systemic antibiotics are generally needed for middle ear infections, which are particularly common in children. However, if there is a long-standing perforation of the eardrum, which divides the outer and middle ears, antibiotic drops can be extremely effective. There is a slight risk that some antibiotic drops could damage the tiny 'hair cells' in the inner ear, and so cause some loss of hearing and dizziness. To minimise this risk, antibiotic drops should be stopped as soon as the infection clears, or if the patient experiences any problems with their balance.
- **Antifungal eardrops** These are used to treat fungal external ear infections.
- **Acetic acid eardrops and sprays** These treat external ear infections by creating an acidic environment that restricts bacterial and fungal growth.
  - **Steroid eardrops** Steroid drops are used alone to ease an allergic skin reaction that is not infected, such as eczema.

Is syringing the ears ever necessary, and can it be harmful?

Wax in the ears serves a useful protective role. Under normal circumstances, the ears are self-cleaning and it is not necessary to remove any wax. Occasionally, however, too much wax builds up. Impacted wax is a major cause of reversible hearing loss in the elderly.

Your doctor will recommend syringing if wax is affecting your hearing, causing discomfort, or preventing an examination of the eardrum. Before syringing, you will be asked to use eardrops to soften the wax: this may make syringing easier. Doctors are reluctant to syringe ears in patients with a history of ear disease or surgery. An inappropriately directed jet of water may force wax deeper into the ear or perforate the eardrum, so removal under the microscope is recommended. Syringing has been thought to cause tinnitus, but the links are unproven; it may be that the beginnings of the tinnitus were present before syringing took place, but it was assumed the syringing was to blame.

ASK THE EXPERT

DRUGS FOR VERTIGO AND TRAVEL SICKNESS

Abnormalities of the vestibular (balance) system result in vertigo (dizziness), and this is often associated with nausea and/or vomiting, particularly when travelling. These symptoms are treated with vestibular sedatives – drugs that act on the brain to suppress inappropriate signals from the inner ear, but can cause drowsiness.
- **Cinnarizine, cyclizine and promethazine** These are tablets which can be obtained over the counter.
- **Prochlorperazine** This is available in sublingual (placed under the tongue but not swallowed) tablet or suppository forms. The suppository or sublingual forms are helpful if vomiting accompanies the dizziness.
- **Betahistine** Often prescribed to patients with recurrent symptoms (for example, those suffering from vertigo, tinnitus and deafness associated with Ménière's disease – a disorder of the inner ear). This medicine is intended for regular long-term use to prevent attacks, rather than to treat acute symptoms of dizziness.

Some people get motion sickness watching a movie on a large screen: the mismatch of signals to the ears, eyes and brain triggers the condition.

DRUGS FOR RHINITIS AND SINUSITIS

The doctor's choice of drop or spray for the nose depends on the cause of the malady, which is generally manifested by rhinitis – inflammation of the nose's mucus membrane.

Allergy is a frequent cause of rhinitis, and often contributes to conditions such as glue ear, asthma and eczema. The first step in treatment is to identify and avoid the allergens that are causing a reaction.

- **Antihistamines** These can be taken topically or systemically. Available without prescription, antihistamine sprays and tablets are very effective when taken for allergic rhinitis. Antihistamine sprays have to be used more frequently than steroid sprays, but many tablet forms are intended to be taken just once a day.
- **Nasal steroid sprays** These reduce the blockage, sneezing and nasal discharge associated with rhinitis, and are particularly effective if the rhinitis is allergic. It is best to take steroids topically, to keep any side effects to a minimum. Doctors will also prescribe these medicines in combination with antibiotics to treat infective sinusitis.
- **Decongestants** These topical medicines work by constricting the blood vessels in the nasal lining, which helps to decongest the nose. They are effective and safe if taken over a few days (no longer than a week) to treat a cold, sinusitis or severe nasal allergy.
- **Sodium cromoglycate** This anti-allergy drug, available in spray form, does not contain steroids, and is therefore often prescribed for children.

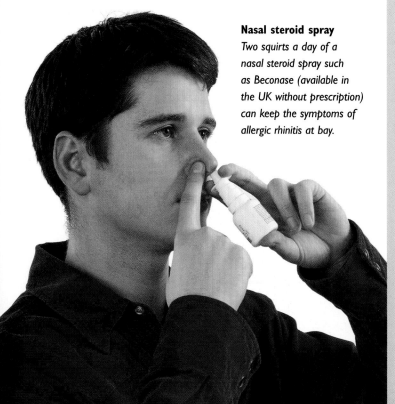

Nasal steroid spray
Two squirts a day of a nasal steroid spray such as Beconase (available in the UK without prescription) can keep the symptoms of allergic rhinitis at bay.

Surgical solutions

Some ear, nose and throat conditions need surgery, much of which is routine and – thanks to modern technology – safer than ever before. Procedures vary, and staff at the ENT clinic are there to talk over any concerns before and after the operation.

BEFORE AN OPERATION

The decision to have an operation is usually made by the patient and the ENT surgeon during an outpatient consultation. Concerns to discuss include:

- If the operation goes well, what are the expected benefits, and what are the chances of a successful long-term outcome?
- What if the operation goes badly? What are the possible complications?
- What is the likely outcome without the operation?

Of course, there are many other factors that will influence the decision to undergo an operation, including:

- Who will actually perform the operation? Although patients will of course be treated by a qualified surgeon, it won't always be the doctor they are accustomed to consulting.
- How long is the wait for the operation?
- How long is the expected hospital stay?
- What is the expected recovery period? Will care be necessary at home after leaving hospital? When will it be possible to resume work?

The pre-admission clinic

It may be difficult for the patient to remember all the necessary information with just one consultation, so many hospitals run a pre-admission clinic, which the patient attends a few weeks before the operation. This allows medical staff to reassess the patient's condition prior to surgery and to complete routine admission tests. It also gives the patient an opportunity to go over the surgical process again and ask more questions.

SPECIAL REQUIREMENTS FOR ENT SURGERY

Many of the operations performed on the ear, nose or throat are delicate procedures, undertaken on tiny structures and with limited access. All this presents the medical team with a special set of challenges.

Minimising bleeding

When operating on tricky, delicate areas within the ears, nose and throat, it is best to keep bleeding to an absolute minimum. Manipulation of the general anaesthetic helps with this, by maintaining blood pressure at a low yet safe level, so that bleeding is minimal.

Special equipment for microscopic surgery

The microscopic size of many structures within the ear, nose and throat necessitates special equipment. The operating microscope and endoscope have dramatically improved the visualisation of these areas, and therefore the quality of surgery carried out. The microscope is routinely used in microlaryngeal (voice box) surgery and all middle ear and mastoid surgery. The endoscope is used in sinus surgery and for examination of the throat and trachea.

Keeping the airway open

Operations on the throat require a close collaboration between the surgeon and anaesthetist, so that the need for access for surgery does not threaten maintenance of the airway. Because general anaesthesia relaxes the throat and chest muscles, the patient's breathing is supported by a tube placed in the throat. This tube maintains a safe passage for air through the throat, and is designed in such a way that it prevents the passage of any foreign matter into the lungs.

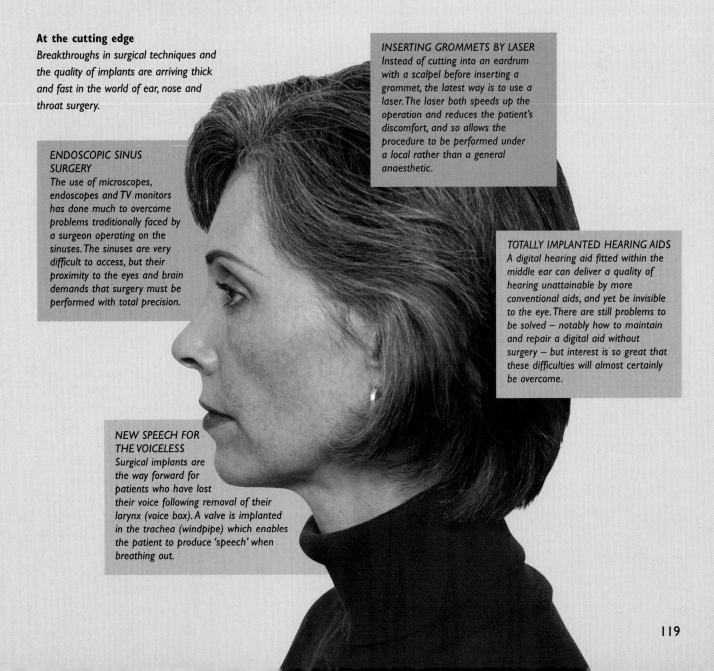

At the cutting edge
Breakthroughs in surgical techniques and the quality of implants are arriving thick and fast in the world of ear, nose and throat surgery.

ENDOSCOPIC SINUS SURGERY
The use of microscopes, endoscopes and TV monitors has done much to overcome problems traditionally faced by a surgeon operating on the sinuses. The sinuses are very difficult to access, but their proximity to the eyes and brain demands that surgery must be performed with total precision.

INSERTING GROMMETS BY LASER
Instead of cutting into an eardrum with a scalpel before inserting a grommet, the latest way is to use a laser. The laser both speeds up the operation and reduces the patient's discomfort, and so allows the procedure to be performed under a local rather than a general anaesthetic.

TOTALLY IMPLANTED HEARING AIDS
A digital hearing aid fitted within the middle ear can deliver a quality of hearing unattainable by more conventional aids, and yet be invisible to the eye. There are still problems to be solved – notably how to maintain and repair a digital aid without surgery – but interest is so great that these difficulties will almost certainly be overcome.

NEW SPEECH FOR THE VOICELESS
Surgical implants are the way forward for patients who have lost their voice following removal of their larynx (voice box). A valve is implanted in the trachea (windpipe) which enables the patient to produce 'speech' when breathing out.

Surgery on the ears

Surgeons perform a range of operations on the ears, the majority of which are to restore or improve impaired hearing. ENT specialists, however, may also carry out cosmetic surgery to improve the profile of the ears.

REMOVING A FOREIGN BODY

Foreign bodies of many different shapes and sizes can get stuck in the ear canal. When removing a foreign body, the doctor takes great care to avoid damaging the eardrum, ossicles (the small bones of the middle ear) or the inner ear. Such damage could lead to hearing loss, tinnitus or vertigo. The foreign body is removed under direct vision, using an operating microscope – if necessary – and a hook, crocodile forceps or suction tube. In most cases involving adults, objects are removed without anaesthetic in the outpatients department, but a child who will wriggle around may need a general anaesthetic.

INSERTING GROMMETS FOR GLUE EAR

Glue ear is the popular name for a condition in which fluid produced by the lining of the middle ear collects behind the eardrum. It occurs most often in children,

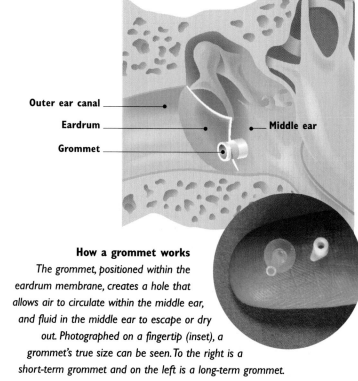

Outer ear canal

Eardrum

Grommet

Middle ear

How a grommet works
The grommet, positioned within the eardrum membrane, creates a hole that allows air to circulate within the middle ear, and fluid in the middle ear to escape or dry out. Photographed on a fingertip (inset), a grommet's true size can be seen. To the right is a short-term grommet and on the left is a long-term grommet.

Were grommets a medical fad?

TALKING POINT

Because most children grow out of glue ear, there has been a move away from inserting grommets. Although specialists agree that glue ear resolves in most children, many feel there is still a case for their use in the 5–10 per cent of children severely affected.

If a child is failing at school or speech is delayed because of deafness, most doctors would recommend inserting grommets to improve hearing. Without grommets, it could be years before the child hears normally and during this time the child will be falling further behind. Also, in some cases, the pressure changes in the middle ear due to the poor eustachian tube function not only cause fluid to collect, but can also damage the eardrum itself, which may become thinned and collapse inwards. This can lead to the formation of cholesteatoma and erosion of the ear's bony ossicles. A grommet inserted at an early stage of these changes can prevent more damage occurring.

usually in both ears. The condition causes partial deafness; if it doesn't resolve, the specialist may carry out an operation called a myringotomy. In this procedure, the eardrum is cut with a microscopic scalpel so that the fluid can escape.

To prevent the incision healing over and the glue ear recurring, a plastic ventilation tube called a grommet is inserted into the incised eardrum. The operation can sometimes be performed under a local anaesthetic, but most patients – especially children – require a general anaesthetic. After insertion, the grommets can cause a mild infection. The resulting discharge is easily treated by cleaning the ear canal and applying antibiotic eardrops.

Short-term grommets are designed to be slowly and painlessly extruded by the eardrum – skin slowly collects under the rim of the tube and pushes the tube out. This takes place over 6–15 months, which is usually long enough for the condition to have resolved. In recurrent cases, doctors may use a non-extruding ventilation tube that is surgically removed 2–3 years later.

REPAIRING A PERFORATED EARDRUM

The eardrum is a thin and delicate structure. It can become perforated as a result of:

- infection;
- direct trauma caused by the insertion of items such as cotton buds;
- indirect trauma, such as a bomb blast or barotrauma from rapid ascent or descent when flying or diving.

Perforations usually heal in days or months without any specific treatment. If this doesn't happen, an operation known as a myringoplasty is often recommended, in which the perforation is closed; nine times out of ten this is successfully achieved. The aim of the operation is to reduce the chance of recurrent infections; sometimes hearing is improved as well.

In a standard myringoplasty, performed under general anaesthetic, the surgeon covers the perforation with a graft of temporalis fascia (connective tissue taken from the temporalis muscle just above the ear). The graft, which is held in place on the eardrum by an absorbable sponge dressing, acts as a scaffold for new blood vessels and skin to grow across. It can take as long as three months for the eardrum to heal fully.

SURGERY ON THE OSSICLES

Hearing loss is sometimes caused by failure of the ossicles – three small bones in the middle ear called the malleus, incus and stapes – to transmit sound from the eardrum to the inner ear. Failure can result from ossicular erosion following chronic middle ear disease, or fracture of the ossicles, or the ossicular chain having fused together (often caused by otosclerosis). An ossiculoplasty or stapedectomy may be recommended to restore hearing.

Ossiculoplasty

In ossiculoplasty, the surgeon lifts the eardrum to reveal the ossicles, then replaces the damaged ossicle with a refashioned one made on the spot from the old, damaged ossicle, or from bone or cartilage taken from elsewhere in the patient's body, or with a synthetic prosthesis. Once the new ossicle is in position, the eardrum is replaced and then held in place with a dressing in the ear canal. It takes 6–12 weeks for the ear to heal fully, and only then can the improvement in hearing be assessed.

Stapedectomy

A stapedectomy involves removing part of the stapes, the innermost of the three ossicles. The surgeon then drills a tiny hole in the immobile stapes footplate in the remaining part of the stapes, and fits a piston-like prosthesis to replace the missing part. This prosthesis takes over the stapes' function of transmitting sound from the incus (the middle ossicle) to the inner ear. While the operation is quoted as having a 98 per cent success rate, it is not without risk; damage to the inner ear can cause hearing loss, tinnitus and/or dizziness. The risk varies from surgeon to surgeon: it is quite legitimate to enquire about a particular surgeon's success rate for this operation.

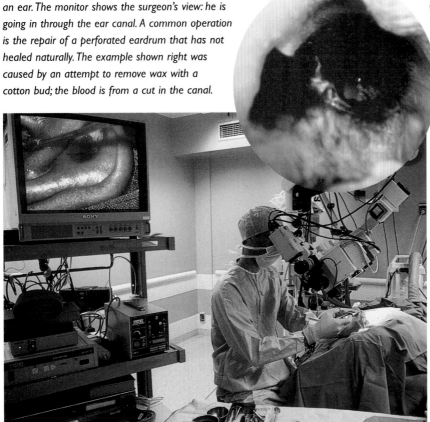

Microsurgery on the ear

A surgeon uses a microscope to perform an operation on an ear. The monitor shows the surgeon's view: he is going in through the ear canal. A common operation is the repair of a perforated eardrum that has not healed naturally. The example shown right was caused by an attempt to remove wax with a cotton bud; the blood is from a cut in the canal.

MASTOID SURGERY

A mastoidectomy is often performed to remove infected matter from the mastoid (the bony protrusion behind the ear and the air space that connects it to the middle ear) and the cavity of the middle ear itself. A typical condition requiring a mastoidectomy is cholesteatoma, which develops when dead, infected skin cells accumulate in the middle ear and mastoid. The surgeon goes in through an incision behind the ear and drills away part of the mastoid bone to expose the diseased area and allow removal of the dead tissue. Often, diseased ossicles must be taken out at the same time; this is likely to cause moderate deafness, if deafness was not present before, but is necessary if the operation is to be successful.

If the surgeon is able to leave the ear canal intact and the eardrum in position (in what is known as the 'canal-wall-up' technique), the possibility of reconstructing the ossicles at a later date remains open, so long as the ear stays free of disease. Sometimes the surgeon has to resort to the more radical 'canal-wall-down' technique, however, in which the canal wall must to be drilled away to remove the diseased area, leading to enlargement of the ear canal and repositioning of the eardrum. Whichever technique is adopted, there is a chance that the condition will return and the ear continue to discharge.

> *One-fifth of the adult population of the UK has enough hearing loss to benefit from the use of a hearing aid.*

HEARING AIDS

Hearing is a complex phenomenon and simply amplifying the surrounding noise electronically is not sufficient. Each aid has to be tailored to the user's own pattern of hearing. Often, an aid must be programmed to amplify high-frequency sounds but not to over-amplify low-frequency sounds, if what the user hears is not to be distorted. A common problem is whistling, due to acoustic feedback resulting from the aid not being correctly fitted in the ear.

Almost all hearing aids now issued are electrical and use an analogue or digital sound system. They are worn behind or inside the ear. For those people who are either unable to wear a standard hearing aid or cannot gain much benefit from one, a surgically implanted hearing aid is often the answer.

Bone-anchored hearing aids

Some patients have diseases of the middle ear that either make it difficult for them to tolerate an earpiece inside the ear, or that block the process of air conduction on which most hearing aids depend. A bone-conducting aid, which transmits sound through the bone behind the ear, can be the solution in such cases. The bone-conducting aid can be worn on a headband, but more convenient is a bone-anchored aid, which is surgically attached to the bone behind the ear. The surgeon implants a titanium screw into the bone of the patient's skull. About six weeks later, the hearing aid is attached to the screw. Bone-anchored aids, introduced in the 1980s, have proved popular, although 5–10 per cent of patients experience healing problems where the screw protrudes through the skin.

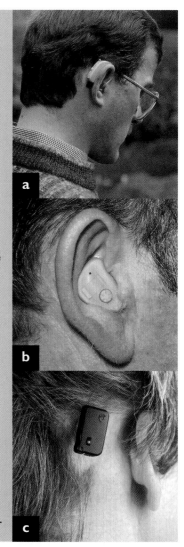

Standard hearing aids

a Sound is picked up by a battery-powered microphone positioned behind the ear, amplified and then transmitted down a transparent plastic tube into a mould that fits into the concha of the outer ear. The aid has a volume control that the user adjusts manually.

b A hearing aid worn in the ear is less visible, but it requires more manual dexterity to place the aid in the ear and to operate the controls. The small dial controls the volume of incoming sound. The flap is the lid to the battery case.

c A bone-anchored hearing aid sits just behind the ear; it transmits sound through the bone behind the ear, bypassing the middle ear. The aid is held in position by a small titanium fixing that has been surgically attached to the patient's skull and protrudes through the skin.

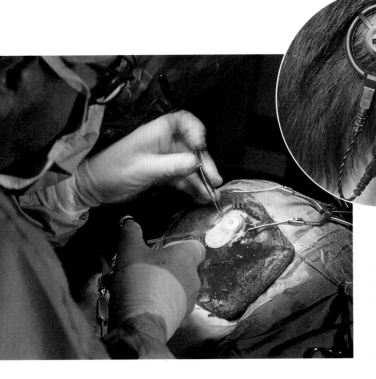

Fitting a cochlear implant
A surgeon places an implant under a flap of skin behind the ear of a patient. Inset: the visible parts of the aid comprise a microphone worn behind the ear that is attached by wires both to a coil held in place above the implant by a magnet and to a speech processor box (not shown here).

Cochlear implants

These devices, in use since the 1970s, provide sound awareness for someone who is profoundly deaf and so beyond the reach of a more traditional hearing aid. A microphone worn behind the ear receives the sound; the signal is then processed in a speech processor box worn on a belt or behind the ear, from where it is transmitted to components internally implanted behind the ear; an electrical signal then travels from the implant to the cochlea via an electrode cable that has been inserted directly into the cochlea of the inner ear.

About half of all cochlear implantees gain a good degree of speech discrimination; some can even use the telephone. However, it can take years of training and practice to get the maximum benefit from the implant.

Totally implantable middle ear hearing aids

Available from the late 1990s, these aids are fitted in the middle ear, where they are attached to the incus (the middle ossicle). The surgeon gains access through the mastoid bone. Hearing results are good when compared to a patient's previous aids, but the implant is costly and requires a complex operation with attendant risks.

SURGERY FOR PROMINENT EARS

A common congenital deformity of the ear is a failure of development of the anti-helical fold (the bend in the wing of the outer ear that moulds an ear so it follows the shape of the head). As a result, the ears appear very prominent, an appearance sometimes referred to as 'bat ears'. In such

cases an operation called a pinnaplasty can deal with the problem. The process involves cutting through the skin behind the ear to reach the cartilage that forms the shape of the ear. Shape is restored by cutting or scoring the cartilage, or bending it to create an anti-helical fold, then holding that position with permanent stitches through the cartilage. A head bandage must be left in place for a week to maintain the new shape and prevent excessive bruising.

OCCASIONAL COMPLICATIONS

Although complications after ear surgery are rare, the inner ear and facial nerve are both vulnerable to accidental damage. Surgeons, aware of this, do their very best to preserve them. The risks, however, must be considered in context – the diseases for which surgery is performed (such as cholesteatoma and chronic infection) can themselves damage the facial nerve or inner ear, or spread infection to the cranial cavity, if they go untreated.

AT THE LEADING EDGE

Digital hearing aids

Digital hearing aids can be worn in or behind the ear. They work by taking a sound signal and converting it into data that is manipulated by a computer in the aid. In this way, sound can be processed precisely and the hearing aid adjusted to suit each user. Digital aids first became available from the NHS in 2001. In general, digital aids perform better than analogue aids. But users of analogue aids convinced that a digital aid is the answer to problems with hearing speech against a noisy background are often not getting the best out of their analogue hearing aid. With time and practice, many users of analogue aids are able to automatically 'screen out' more obtrusive background noises than they could to begin with.

Removing nasal polyps

The latest and most complete way of removing nasal polyps is by means of endoscopic sinus surgery, in which cutting-edge surgical instruments enable a surgeon to take out polyps entirely, with minimal trauma to the nose itself.

Nasal polyps tend to occur in patients with rhinitis; rare in children, they are more common in men than women. They are normally benign, resulting only in some loss of smell and/or blocked breathing. When they are removed, it is generally because they form an obstruction within the nose. Rarely, a benign or malignant sinus tumour can create polyps, usually on one side of the nose.

Nasal polyps are treated either with steroid medications or with surgery, and often a combination of both. The surgeon usually requests a CT scan of the sinuses to determine the extent of the disease and to help plan any operations.

The simplest surgical procedure is an intranasal polypectomy – removal of polyps from the nasal passages, under local or general anaesthetic. The operation improves breathing and, to a variable degree, the patient's sense of smell, but there is a possibility that the polyps will return.

Endoscopic sinus surgery

More extensive surgery removes the polyps not just from the nose but also from the sinuses where they originate, thus decreasing the chances of recurrence. Endoscopic sinus surgery (ESS) enables the surgeon to follow the disease into the sinuses and remove it entirely.

Endoscopic sinus surgery has largely replaced the more traditional sinus operations, in which surgical cuts were made on the face or under the upper lip. Disadvantages of traditional 'open' sinus surgery include external scarring, greater bruising and discomfort, and more bleeding. However, traditional 'open' surgery is still regarded as the most efficient option in some circumstances, such as when a tumour must be removed from the sinuses.

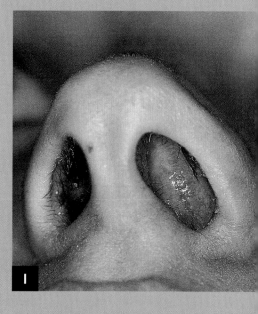

The surgical procedure

1 The nasal polyp that is to be cut out is clearly visible and totally blocking the patient's nostril. It originates in the maxillary sinus, and will be removed using minimally invasive techniques known as endoscopic sinus surgery (ESS). As soon as the patient has been anaesthetised, the nasal lining is prepared for surgery with medications that decongest the mucous membrane. This helps to improve visibility and reduce bleeding.

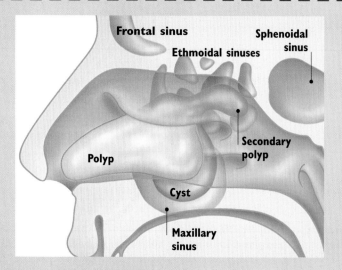

Frontal sinus
Sphenoidal sinus
Ethmoidal sinuses
Polyp
Secondary polyp
Cyst
Maxillary sinus

Polyps within the nose and sinuses

Nasal polyps are round, smooth, soft, swollen, semi-translucent structures which appear singly or in a cluster that can resemble a small bunch of grapes. Polyps originate in the swollen or prolapsed lining of one of the paranasal sinuses, to which they are attached by a stalk. They extend into the nasal cavity and, often, down one or both nostrils. They most commonly develop in the ethmoidal sinuses, a collection of air-filled spaces within the ethmoid bone (between the nose and the floor of the cavity containing the brain). Sometimes a polyp is attached to a cyst positioned at the opening of one of the maxillary sinuses.

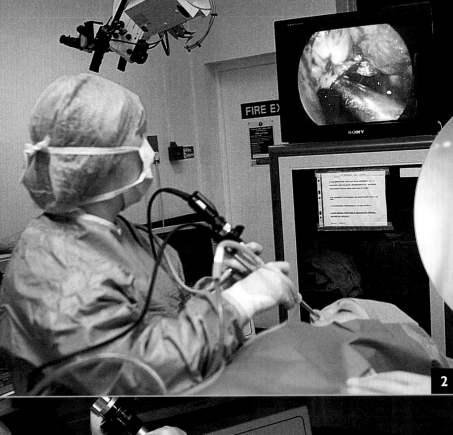

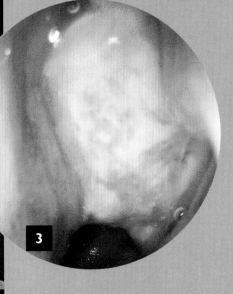

3

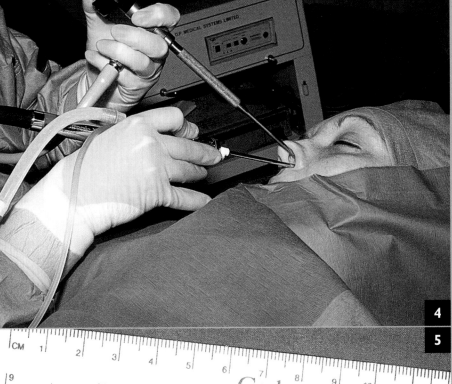

2

4

5

CM 1 2 3 4 5 6 7 8 9 10 11 12

Codman

2 By inserting a rigid 4mm endoscope into the nostril in which the polyp is growing, the surgeon can clearly visualise the inside of the nose. The tip of the endoscope is fitted with a fibreoptic light that illuminates the operation site and a high resolution camera that transmits an image of the site to a large viewing monitor. Throughout the operation the surgeon is able to see the site and monitor the progress of the operation on the screen.

3 A secondary polyp in the back of the nose, with surrounding infection, is identified and displayed on the monitor.

4 Working parallel to the endoscope (held in her left hand) the surgeon can introduce a variety of instruments into the same nostril. Specialised angled instruments allow access to all the nasal sinuses, but here a powered debrider is being used to cut and aspirate away targeted tissue while leaving the surrounding mucous membrane untouched. The suction tubing keeps the operation site clear.

5 The main body of the polyp, now removed, is a surprising 4cm (1.5in) long. It is attached to a large cyst which was removed from the left maxillary sinus.

Nose and sinus surgery

A variety of conditions affecting the nose and sinuses require surgery, from congenital defects to severe cases of rhinitis. Microscopes and endoscopes have revolutionised surgical procedures in these areas, making them safer and more effective than ever before.

TREATING RHINITIS

Most cases of rhinitis – inflammation of the lining of the nose – are treated with medication (see page 118). Some cases can require surgical intervention however, as with rhinitis due to chronic swelling of the turbinates (ridges covered with mucous membrane) within the nasal cavity. A local anaesthetic is applied and a laser or electrocautery is used to reduce the swelling.

CORRECTING A DEVIATED SEPTUM

The nasal septum is the cartilage and bone partition that separates the nostrils. A deviated – or twisted – septum reduces airflow through the nasal passages; it generally affects one side more than the other. A deviated septum may be congenital or result from an injury such as a blow to the nose. Surgery under general anaesthetic should solve the problem. There are two main types of operation.

- **Submucous resection of the nasal septum** Deviated bone and cartilage is removed from under the lining of the septum, and then the lining is replaced.
- **Septoplasty** In this procedure, a minimal amount of the distorted cartilage and bone is removed and the remaining parts are realigned in the centre.

Nasal-septal perforation

There should be no internal communication between the two sides of the nose. Occasionally, a connection between the two sides – a nasal-septal perforation – occurs, but this rarely causes problems. If it does, graft techniques are used to close it.

Aesthetic nasal surgery

Rhinoplasty is the most common aesthetic surgical procedure in the UK. A rhinoplasty reshapes or rebalances the nose and can have a dramatic impact on a person's appearnace and self-esteem. The majority of requests are for nasal reduction. Most aesthetic surgery is performed internally via the nostrils, so there is no visible scarring.

Choosing to have nose surgery is a personal decision and not one to make lightly. A reputable surgeon will be able to advise on what can be achieved in each individual

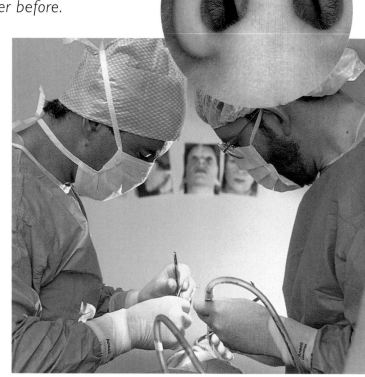

Plastic surgery on the nose
Rhinoplasty – surgery to alter the shape or internal structure of the nose – is performed either to correct a problem which affects the nose's ability to function properly, such as a twisted septum (shown top, between the two nostrils), or for purely aesthetic reasons (above).

case. Anyone performing such surgery should be a consultant surgeon specialising in facial plastic surgery, and on the Specialist Register of the GMC.

SURGERY FOR RECURRENT SINUSITIS

In some patients prone to recurrent sinus infections, the connecting passages between the nose and sinuses are too narrow. To enlarge these openings, and improve drainage through the natural pathways into the nose, the technique known as functional endoscopic sinus surgery (FESS) is employed. By using an endoscope to view the sinus openings on a monitor, a surgeon is able to enlarge the sinus openings, using a cutting tool introduced into the nasal cavity via a nostril. FESS leaves no external scars and can be performed under local or general anaesthetic.

Throat surgery

The throat forms a passageway through which you breathe, eat and speak. Surgery on this vital part of the body is a common procedure for the staff of an ENT unit, with operations ranging from routine tonsillectomies to life-saving tracheostomies.

REMOVING THE TONSILS

The tonsils are at the back of the throat, positioned opposite each other, and attached to the side walls; their surgical removal is known as a tonsillectomy. They are made of the lymphoid tissue that forms part of the body's defence against infection. But because there is sufficient lymphoid tissue elsewhere in the upper respiratory tract to substitute for what has been removed, patients usually develop fewer throat infections after a tonsillectomy rather than more, as might logically be expected. This is because a major focus of infection has been removed.

When is a tonsillectomy recommended?

• **Acute tonsillitis** Tonsils can become subject to a series of attacks of acute tonsillitis, caused by repeated infection. Symptoms include a prolonged, severe sore throat with swollen, inflamed tonsils, plus difficulty in swallowing, fever and a general feeling of being ill. A tonsillectomy – suggested in severe cases – won't prevent another sore throat but will bring an end to these acute attacks.

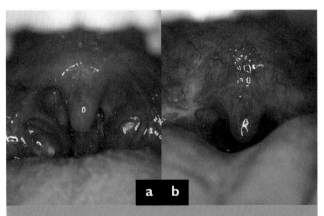

Before and after a tonsillectomy

a A child shows symptoms of severe tonsillitis, with swollen tonsils, whitish pus and a white-coated tongue. The cause is a streptococcal infection,

b This 20-year-old had a tonsillectomy ten years ago. A scar left by the operation is still visible where one of the tonsils used to be.

• **Enlarged tonsils** Children with enlarged tonsils can find it difficult to sleep properly because the tonsils obstruct their breathing. To improve the breathing, a surgeon may recommend removal of the tonsils, and often the adenoids as well, if they too are enlarged.
• **Draining a quinsy** A peritonsillar abscess, also known as a quinsy, develops when pus – produced as part of the body's reaction to an infection – collects between a tonsil and the muscles of the throat. It may be possible to drain the abscess using a needle or by means of a cut made under local anaesthetic. In some cases the surgeon will recommend a tonsillectomy, to be performed either at the time of draining the abscess or after it has settled.
• **Removal of a tumour** Very occasionally, a single enlarged tonsil is a sign of a tumour. This may be a lymphoma (a tumour originating in lymphatic tissue) or a squamous carcinoma (a tumour originating in the lining of the throat and most commonly occurring in smokers).

The operation and afterwards

A tonsillectomy is performed under general anaesthetic. With the mouth held open by a retractor, the tonsils are carefully dissected and removed. Bleeding is stopped with electrocautery or by surgical ties. The patient generally leaves hospital the day after the operation, with a sore throat that usually lasts about 7 to 10 days.

REMOVING THE ADENOIDS

The adenoids form another collection of lymphoid tissue, similar to that in the tonsils. They are found in the region behind the nose called the nasopharynx. They generally shrink in size during adolescence, and so children will often outgrow any adenoidal problems. However, some conditions need to be dealt with sooner rather than later – in these cases the solution is often an adenoidectomy.

When is an adenoidectomy recommended?

- **Enlarged adenoids** The passage of air through the eustachian tube that connects the ear to the throat can be obstructed by enlarged adenoids. When this regularly disrupts a child's sleep, surgery may be the answer.
- **Middle ear infections** There is increasing evidence that removing the adenoids may reduce the duration of middle ear infections such as 'glue ear'. The operation is often combined with the insertion of grommets.
- **Infected adenoids** Until recently, children with rhinitis coupled with a general feeling of being unwell were likely to be diagnosed as having chronically infected adenoids, for which the cure was to have the adenoids cut out. Nowadays, these symptoms are often diagnosed as an allergic response that is more effectively treated by other means. A deep-seated infection of the adenoids is still sometimes treated by their removal, however.

The operation

An adenoidectomy is performed under general anaesthetic and usually takes less than 15 minutes. Operating through the mouth with the aid of a mirror, the surgeon shaves away layers of adenoidal tissue. Electrocautery keeps bleeding to a minimum. The tonsils are often removed at the same time, but if the adenoids alone are excised, the patient's throat is much less sore afterwards.

FOREIGN BODIES IN THE THROAT

All sorts of objects can lodge in the throat – small bones, lumps of gristle, nuts and coins are common examples. If these don't clear by themselves, they have to be removed surgically. The procedure depends on what the object is and where it is stuck. As well as being swallowed, foreign bodies can be inhaled and lodge in the larynx (voice box), trachea (windpipe) or bronchi (airways from the trachea to the lungs). A small bone lodged in a tonsil is easily removed with forceps after a spray of local anaesthetic. Removing an object further down the throat often

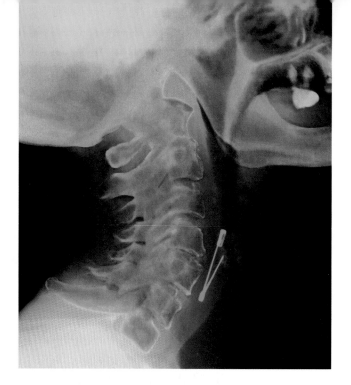

Stuck in the throat
This side view X-ray shows a safety pin, accidentally swallowed. Sharp foreign bodies form a particular danger when lodged in the gullet (oesophagus), because they can perforate the oesophageal walls.

requires a general anaesthetic. After locating the object by means of an X-ray and/or a flexible endoscope passed down the throat, the surgeon retrieves it with grasping forceps attached to an endoscope or rigid bronchoscope.

REMOVING VOCAL NODULES AND POLYPS

Nodules – almost always benign – appear on the vocal cords in pairs, one on each cord. These tiny, hardened, grey-white lumps develop on the cords of people – often singers or teachers – who habitually overuse their voices and so strain their vocal cords. It is generally hoarseness that sends them to the doctor. Treatment involves resting the voice, speech therapy and avoiding irritants such as cigarette smoke. With this treatment the nodules will shrink and hopefully disappear. If the nodules fail to shrink sufficiently, or are very large to begin with, they are removed surgically. Viewing a magnified image of the vocal cords, the surgeon uses a laryngoscope with a carbon dioxide laser or scalpel to remove the nodes.

One or more polyps on the cords appear as smooth, rounded swellings. Like nodules, they are generally benign. The symptoms, causes and initial treatment are usually the same as for nodules. However, most polyps end up having to be removed surgically (following procedures similar to those used when removing nodules). Polyps and nodules can return if the patient does not modify poor voice habits and strains the voice again.

TRACHEOSTOMY

Tracheostomy is a procedure that creates an opening in the neck into which a tube is inserted that enters the trachea, below the larynx and vocal cords. The aim is to maintain the passage of air to the lungs. The patient breathes in and out through the open tracheostomy tube. A tracheostomy tube may be inserted because:

- the airway is obstructed higher up;
- the patient must use an artificial ventilator for help with breathing, all or part of the time;
- the patient has problems with fluids entering the airway from the throat;
- the airway opening has to be rerouted as part of a major operation involving the head and neck.

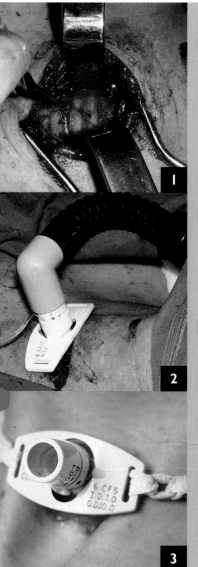

The tracheostomy tube

1 Having made an incision in the skin of the patient's neck, the surgeon cuts through to the trachea (windpipe) to form an opening known as a stoma, and then inserts a short length of tube to maintain the opening.

2 Once the tracheostomy tube is in place it can be attached to a ventilator which administers the general anaesthetic during an operation.

3 When the tracheostomy tube is open, as here, air enters and leaves the lungs via the tube. When the tube is shut, air enters and leaves the lungs via the nose or mouth. To maintain the stoma, the tube must be kept in place. To reverse the tracheostomy, the tube is simply replaced by a dressing and the opening begins to close over within a few days.

Can you speak after a tracheostomy?

Breathing through a tracheostomy tube means that air is diverted before it reaches the vocal cords. Since a stream of air is needed for the vocal cords to work, a patient with an open tracheostomy tube can't use the vocal cords to produce the sounds needed for speech. However, most patients who undergo a tracheostomy can manage to speak satisfactorily. Some patients have a tube that is covered most of the time; for them, speech is not a problem, Others can cover the opening whenever they want to speak. For others, the solution depends on the nature of the problem. For example, someone with a tracheostomy because the airway is only partially obstructed may be able to breathe with the help of a smaller-than-normal tube, so that with each out breath some air exits via the tube and some passes through the vocal cords.

ASK THE EXPERT

When the airway is obstructed

The airway can become obstructed by a foreign body or as a result of injury, an infection or a disease such as cancer. The airway can only be completely blocked for a few minutes before brain damage starts to take place, so a tracheostomy may need to be carried out as an emergency bypass of the blockage. More often, however, there is a gradual onset to the airway obstruction, allowing time to plan a tracheostomy in advance.

When the patient is dependent on a ventilator

A tracheostomy is often performed on patients who cannot breathe naturally and require artificial ventilation (pumping of air into the lungs by a machine) either all or part of the time. If the patient has not had a tracheostomy, a ventilation tube is passed down the larynx and into the upper trachea via the mouth or nose. This is so uncomfortable that the patient usually has to be sedated while artificial ventilation takes place.

Attaching the ventilation tube to a tracheostomy tube instead brings a number of benefits: the patient can breathe without sedation; it becomes easier to wean the patient from a ventilator; and the airway is no longer in danger of becoming scarred or permanently narrowed by prolonged use of the ventilation tube.

Removing head and neck tumours

The surgery performed on head and neck tumours (principally cancers of the throat, mouth or tongue) is often life-saving. Specialists are on hand every step of the way to help patients through the operation and support them on their journey back to health.

LOCATION AND TREATMENT

Each year, about 3000 patients in the UK develop cancer of the head and neck. Most cases are of a type known as squamous cell carcinoma, principally caused by smoking. Cancers can occur anywhere in the lining of the mouth, throat or larynx (voice box), and treatment depends on the location, size and spread of the tumour. In general, squamous cell carcinomas first spread from the primary site to the lymph glands in the neck; in approximately five in a hundred cases, they spread to more distant regions of the body, such as the lungs, liver or bones. The recommended treatment is usually surgery, radiotherapy or a combination of both. In certain instances, chemotherapy may also be recommended.

> **Two-thirds of the people diagnosed with laryngeal cancer are treated early enough to preserve the voice box.**

SURGERY ON THE VOCAL CORDS

One of the most common lesions is a tumour of the vocal cords within the larynx. These are usually spotted early, because even a very small growth will make the patient's voice sound hoarse. Tumours may need removal using micro-surgical techniques, often performed with a laser. A relatively good quality of voice is usually regained following surgery. An alternative treatment for small vocal cord tumours is radiotherapy.

LARYNGECTOMY

Larger tumours of the larynx, or those that recur after radiotherapy, require more extensive surgery. This may mean the partial or total removal of the larynx – an operation referred to as a laryngectomy. A partial laryngectomy may be performed by means of an endoscopic laser technique, or via an incision in the neck. If the latter course is taken, a temporary tracheostomy is often necessary. If the entire larynx has to be cut out, the tracheostomy is permanent. Following a total laryngectomy, therefore, the patient is unable to speak and must breathe through the opening in their neck created by the tracheostomy (see page 129).

Regaining speech after a laryngectomy

The vast majority of patients regain some form of speech following a laryngectomy, and there are several ways they can achieve this, with the help of regular practice under the supervision of a specially trained speech therapist.

- **A speech valve** This usually produces the best results as far as voice quality is concerned. The valve is implanted at the back of the windpipe. A patient who wants to speak places a finger over the open tracheostomy tube and breathes out; air

A speech therapist at work
A patient who has undergone a tracheostomy as part of a laryngectomy, and so has lost her vocal cords, learns to talk again using oesophageal speech, with the help of a speech therapist.

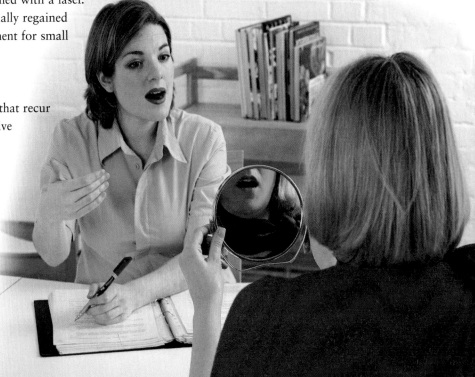

that would normally exit via the tube passes into the throat and through the valve, which resonates in a similar way to the vocal cords.

- **Oesophageal speech** The basic idea is to swallow air and then regurgitate it to produce speech; in fact, oesophageal speech resembles an energetic form of burping. Quite intelligible speech can be produced by this method, but sentences often have to be kept short.

- **An electrolarynx** This is an electrical source of vibration. Holding the battery operated device against the neck, the patient speaks in a normal manner and the device translates this into an electronic, monotone voice. The speech can be understood but has a metallic, tinny quality that some patients don't feel comfortable with.

SURGERY ON THE TONGUE AND PHARYNX

Tumours of the tongue and pharynx (the muscular tube leading from the back of the nose and mouth to the top of the oesophagus) are often removed along with part or all of the surrounding area. This can have a dramatic effect on the patient's ability to swallow. Small operations may produce only a temporary problem; more extensive procedures can necessitate careful reconstruction of the swallowing passage, using muscles from the chest wall or pieces of the intestine or stomach. Once healed, these can work as well as the original passage structure.

Learning to swallow again

Throughout the healing process, the patient is fed through a tube, which is usually passed up the nose or directly into the stomach through the abdomen. While in hospital, patients are shown how to use the feeding tube and associated equipment, so that they can manage them at home. Regular sessions with a speech therapist – also an expert on swallowing – help the patient to recover the ability to swallow. Following a swallowing assessment, which may take the form of a video X-ray examination or an endoscopic guided examination (see page 111) of the swallowing mechanism, the therapist will advise on manoeuvres and exercises that will help a patient regain the ability to swallow, and do without the feeding tube.

Cancer in the lymph glands
In this coloured single photon CT scan of a head, lymph glands invaded by cells that are cancerous show up yellow and red.

SURGERY FOR CANCEROUS LYMPH NODES

Foreign swellings that have spread to the lymph glands of the neck can be treated by surgical removal or radiotherapy. The choice of treatment is based on a number of factors. The site and size, as well as the type of treatment given for the initial tumour, are important. For example, larger lumps in the neck are often treated surgically. The tumour pathology report will influence the decision, as will the number of neck glands affected, and whether the tumour has spread outside the lymph glands.

Neck dissection

An operation in which the lymph glands are removed from one side of the neck is known as a neck dissection. The extent of the neck dissection depends on the location and size of the primary tumour. There are about 200 lymph glands in the neck; in a typical neck dissection, between 30 and 50 glands might be removed.

The operation is performed through an incision in the neck. Although great care is taken not to damage any nerves, blood vessels or muscles, this can be unavoidable. For instance, if the major nerve to the shoulder (called the spinal accessory nerve) is affected by the disease, it may have to be cut. This causes some stiffness in the shoulders and weakness in the muscles used to shrug the shoulder, and is followed with physiotherapy. In some cases the large muscle of the neck, the sternocleidomastoid, may be removed. This generally changes the contour of the neck, leaving a hollowed-out profile on one side.

A LUMP IN THE THYROID GLAND

A lump in the neck is sometimes, in fact, a lump in the thyroid gland. This is an endocrine gland that manufactures and secretes hormones into the bloodstream. It consists of two lobes on either side of the Adam's apple at the top of the trachea, connected by a narrow band of thyroid tissue known as the isthmus.

The lump or lumps may be cancerous or benign. To find out, the doctor will begin by ordering a fine-needle aspiration cytology (FNAC) test (see page 112), plus an ultrasound scan. When the diagnosis is cancer within the thyroid, a surgeon will generally remove part or all of the thyroid gland; the function of the gland is replaced by the patient taking thyroid hormone – generally in pill form – every day for the rest of their life. Follow-up treatment to eliminate remaining cancer cells depends on the type and extent of the cancer, but may include doses of radioactive iodine and/or external beam radiotherapy. Radioactive iodine is either swallowed or injected into a vein in the arm; only thyroid cells – both cancerous and healthy – will absorb the iodine and so inevitably receive a high dose of radiation as well.

A benign lump is also often removed, at least partially, because of the risk of it compressing any of the crucial structures in the neck, especially the trachea.

A lump may be a symptom of the thyroid gland being overactive and producing too much thyroid hormone. Removing part of the thyroid was once the most common treatment, but this has been largely replaced by the use of radioactive iodine and various drugs to bring the amount of hormones produced down to a normal level.

THE COMBINED HEAD AND NECK CLINIC

At some point, a patient with a head or neck tumour will probably be referred to a special combined clinic for head and neck complaints. Here the patient will see a variety of specialists including surgeons, oncologists (specialists in the treatment of tumours), specialist nurses, speech therapists, radiotherapists, dietitians and physiotherapists. Each specialist contributes to designing a total treatment programme for the patient, taking into account the nature, size and site of the tumour.

- **Clinical nurse specialists** Not only can these nurses help with pain control, dressings and so forth, but they are a key point of contact for a patient if new problems arise. They may well have received training as Macmillan nurses (specialists in cancer treatment and care).
- **Physiotherapists** Shoulder and neck pain and stiffness are common following head and neck surgery and physiotherapy can often help.
- **Dietitians** Maintaining a healthy diet and body weight is difficult when the ability to swallow is limited – perhaps so limited that the patient can only take liquids. The dietitian works out the best diet for each patient and in

what form it's best taken. Patients on tube feeding need guidance on how often and for how long they must feed via the tube to get the nutrients they need.

EXTERNAL BEAM RADIOTHERAPY

External beam radiotherapy is a key treatment for tumours of the head and neck. This involves controlled doses of ionising radiation which slow or destroy the development of abnormal cells in diseased tissue. It is given either on its own, before surgery or after surgery, and is usually carried out over six weeks, with a patient attending the clinic most weekdays.

Information gained from scans and examinations of the tumour with an endoscope will have determined which regions to irradiate. During the patient's first visit, treatments are discussed and a mould is made of the patient's head and neck. At each subsequent visit, the patient's head is fixed in position by a clear plastic mask and a very precise dose of radiation is delivered to the area that requires treatment.

To reduce side effects, the amount of radiation delivered to the area surrounding the tumour is kept to an absolute minimum. Despite this, some patients who undergo head and neck radiotherapy complain of a permanently dry mouth and throat; a troublesome feeling that can last for months or even years. This is caused by radiation disturbing the salivary glands that keep the mouth and throat moist. An artificial salivary product will ease this side effect, as will frequent sips of water.

A patient receives radiotherapy
A custom-made plastic mask is used during every dose of radiotherapy to ensure the patient's head is always in exactly the same position, so that precisely the same spot is exposed to the radiation every time.

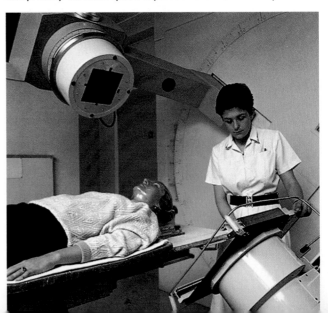

A TO Z

OF DISEASES AND DISORDERS

This section gives information on the main illnesses and medical conditions that can affect the ears, nose and throat.

This index is arranged alphabetically and each entry is structured in a similar way:

What are the causes?

What are the symptoms?

How is it diagnosed?

What are the treatment options?

What is the outlook?

ACOUSTIC NEUROMA

A benign tumour on the nerve that carries balance and hearing from the inner ear to the brain.

An acoustic neuroma (also known as a vestibular schwannoma) is a growth on part of the nerve which is involved in balance and hearing. The growth is benign – it is not a cancer – but because of its proximity to the brain it can have serious effects if it grows to be very large.

What are the symptoms?

The most common symptom is a gradual loss of hearing in one ear. Other less common symptoms include:
• tinnitus;
• balance problems;
• facial pain, numbness or tingling.
Very large tumours may cause headache, double vision, facial paralysis and (rarely) drowsiness.

How is it diagnosed?

A hearing test is often the first investigation. This will show up any hearing loss in the affected ear. An MRI scan of the head (p.115) is then the best investigation to detect an acoustic neuroma. For patients who are unable to undergo MRI scanning a CT scan may be appropriate, with or without tests of auditory function called brainstem response audiometry.

Severe claustrophobia or a surgical implant such as a pacemaker may make a patient unsuitable for MRI scanning.

What are the treatment options?

Each case is assessed on its own merits, taking into consideration factors such as the size and position of the tumour, the age and general health of the patient and the patient's preferences for treatment.

Surgery aims for total removal of the tumour with as little damage to surrounding brain tissue and nerves as possible. Recovery from surgery can take up to three months and some degree of hearing loss or facial nerve paralysis is not uncommon. However, once removed totally the tumour is unlikely to return.

Stereotactic radiosurgery, or the gamma knife, is a form of radiotherapy in which the beams are focused specifically on the small area of tumour. In this way, radiation to surrounding tissues is minimised. This is suitable only for smaller tumours, and in some cases the tumour may not disappear completely but may shrink or its growth may be stopped.

Where the tumour grows very slowly, it may be worth monitoring the tumour with regular scans before treatment is considered, since the risks of treatment can be greater than the problems the tumour is causing.

What is the outlook?

Acoustic neuromas tend to be slow-growing tumours, so decisions about treatment do not have to be rushed. Intensive rehabilitation after surgery will get most people back to a full and active life.

BAROTRAUMA

The effect that changes in atmospheric pressure have on the ear.

Changes in air pressure, such as when flying or scuba diving, can cause ear pain and hearing problems.

What is the cause?

Barotrauma is caused by a failure to equalise the pressure of the middle ear with the pressure of the external surroundings, due to poor eustachian tube function. The eustachian tube, which runs from the back of the nose to the middle ear, normally allows air into and out of the ear to keep the pressure equal to atmospheric pressure. This produces the popping sensation we normally feel in the ears with pressure changes.

What are the symptoms?

As atmospheric pressure changes, for example on descent in an aeroplane, the ear becomes painful and fails to pop to clear. Hearing is usually muffled. These symptoms often resolve spontaneously within hours or days, but may persist, particularly if the barotrauma has caused fluid to collect in the middle ear (an effusion).

How is it diagnosed?

Examination of the ear using an otoscope may reveal fluid or blood behind the eardrum. This may be confirmed by a hearing test and a test to measure the movement of the eardrum and middle ear pressure, known as tympanometry (p.108).

What are the treatment options?

Prevention can be important for those who are known to have suffered problems in the past. People should avoid flying if they have a severe cold or upper respiratory tract infection. Sucking sweets or sipping a drink during take-off and descent can help, as can nasal decongestants taken before the journey.

Divers should be trained to equalise middle ear pressure during a dive, and should avoid diving if they are unable to do this. A myringotomy, making a small hole in the eardrum, to drain any residual fluid can treat persistent deafness. A grommet (p.120) can be inserted if necessary, for example in frequent flyers with recurrent problems.

BROKEN NOSE
A fracture of the nasal bones.

A common result of a blow to the nose, such as may occur through assault, car accident or sporting injury.

What are the symptoms?
Once the bruising and swelling caused by the injury disappear, there may be no obvious sign of a fracture. The nose may remain tender to touch for a few weeks, and there may be a change in the shape of the nose.

How is it diagnosed?
Most fractures are diagnosed by talking to the patient and physically examining the nose. X-rays are required only if other injuries of the bones of the face are suspected, or if evidence of the fracture is required for legal purposes, where criminal proceedings may occur for example.

What are the treatment options?
If there is no deformity of the nose after the swelling has gone down, usually about one week after receiving the injury, no treatment is necessary. If there is an obvious change in the shape of the nose, manipulation of the bones under general anaesthetic may be necessary. This is usually performed within two weeks of the injury before the bones have fully set. If the shape cannot be corrected by simple manipulation, cosmetic surgery, or rhinoplasty, may be required.

CANCER OF THE LARYNX
Cancer affecting the area of the throat around and including the voice box.

In the West this is the commonest cancer affecting the head and neck; there are some 2000 cases each year in the UK.

What is the cause?
Certain factors are known to trigger the changes in cells that lead to cancer, in particular smoking and heavy alcohol consumption.

What are the symptoms?
A hoarse voice, which does not get better, is the commonest and often the only symptom. Other symptoms include difficulty swallowing and breathing, pain in the throat or ear, and sometimes a lump in the neck.

How is it diagnosed?
The larynx can be examined in the ENT clinic either using a mirror, or a flexible endoscope. If a suspicious area is seen, a biopsy needs to be taken; this is performed under a general anaesthetic. Scans of the throat and neck, along with the biopsy findings, will help to determine the most suitable treatment.

What are the treatment options?
Treatment depends upon the exact site and size of the tumour, on whether there is any spread to the neck glands, and on the health and preferences of the patient.

Radiotherapy is appropriate for some smaller tumours. On average, a course of treatment lasts six weeks. It is also sometimes given after surgical treatment, if it is felt there is a risk that the tumour may recur.

Surgery can vary from localised treatment, such as laser surgery for small tumours, to more extensive operations, such as laryngectomy, for larger tumours. Laryngectomy involves removing the voice box and part of the windpipe, leaving a small hole or stoma in the neck for breathing.

If the tumour is very large, part of the top end of the oesophagus may also need to be removed and tissue is then taken from other parts of the body to repair this. Rehabilitation from such surgery involves relearning swallowing and speech. Despite the surgical removal of the voice box many patients achieve an excellent 'voice' with the help of a speech therapist.

If the disease has spread to the neck, surgery may be required to remove the lymph nodes; this is usually performed at the same time.

What is the outlook?
Five-year survival for this cancer is 50–60 per cent. The outlook for individual patients depends on the extent of the tumour at the time of diagnosis. At initial diagnosis, 95 per cent of patients will be treatable, although not all

Medicine, surgery, radiotherapy and chemotherapy all control symptoms and ease cancer pain.

curable. Patients who have had treatment are followed up closely at regular intervals to detect any sign of the return of the cancer so that further treatment can be planned quickly if it should become necessary.

CANCER OF THE NASOPHARYNX
A tumour of the area at the back of the nose.

The nasopharynx is the area at the back of the nose above the palate. Although cancer can occur in people of any race, in this area it is most common among people of Chinese origin. There may be a genetic element to the disease, but modifiable risk factors include avoiding salted fish (an oriental staple from infancy) and fermented foods.

What are the symptoms?
Many patients have no symptoms until the tumour is very large. Many complain of nasal blockage, nosebleeds or a lump in the neck. The tumour may block the eustachian tube, leading to a build up of fluid and deafness.

How is it diagnosed?
The nasopharynx can be examined in the ENT clinic using a mirror or an endoscope. If there is any suspicion that there is a tumour present, a biopsy is performed under general anaesthetic, usually in the operating theatre. Scans can be useful in planning treatment.

What are the treatment options?
Radiotherapy with chemotherapy is the treatment of choice. Surgery is occasionally necessary to remove the neck glands, if the disease has spread to them.

What is the outlook?
Depending on the extent of the disease when a patient is first diagnosed, five-year survival can be up to 90 per cent.

DEVIATED NASAL SEPTUM
A bent or misshapen septum – the partition in the nose that divides it into left and right cavities.

What is the cause?
The septum may become bent following an accident or during growth of the nose in childhood.

What are the symptoms?
The nose will feel blocked on the narrower side, and the deviation may sometimes cause external twisting of the shape of the nose.

What is the treatment?
If treatment is required to relieve the blockage, surgery is indicated. The operation is called a septoplasty or sub-mucus resection of the septum. The septum is made of cartilage and bone, and this can be straightened from inside the nose by removing some of the tissue and repositioning the rest. In the UK, this is commonly performed under a general anaesthetic.

What is the outlook?
Recovery from surgery is usually quick. For the first week to ten days there is a little discomfort in the nose, described by most people as feeling like a blockage or pressure. There is a small chance of infection in the nose for a week after surgery – after all, the nose is not the cleanest of areas – which can lead to bleeding, known as secondary haemorrhage. This does not seem to be prevented by giving prophylactic antibiotics, but an infection should respond well to a course of treatment.

Although surgery to correct a deviated septum requires a general anaesthetic, patients can usually go home the same day.

The nose should be healed and the patient able to resume normal activities within two weeks of surgery.

EPIGLOTTITIS
Inflammation of the epiglottis due to infection.

The epiglottis is a leaf-shaped structure in the throat that helps to close the airway during swallowing to prevent food and drink going down the 'wrong way' into the lungs. Inflammation of this structure is called epiglottitis.

What is the cause?
Infection is caused by bacteria and occurs most commonly in children between 2 and 6 years old, but it can occur in adults. The pattern of incidence is changing due to the introduction of the Hib vaccine.

What are the symptoms?
The infection may occur at any time of year but is more common in the winter. The first symptom is usually a sore throat. The epiglottis becomes swollen and the pain

TALKING
POINT

Hib vaccination has virtually eradicated epiglottitis

By far the commonest bacterium causing epiglottitis, as well as one of the strains of meningitis, is the *Haemophilus influenzae*. Vaccination against this organism, introduced in the UK in 1992 and given at two, three and four months of age, has brought about a dramatic 96 per cent reduction in the number of cases of epiglottitis in the very young. Uptake is still important, however, as there are other organisms that can cause the condition, especially in adults, and there is a small pool of children who for various reasons have not been vaccinated.

becomes more severe so that even swallowing saliva is difficult and the patient drools. The voice becomes muffled, and as swelling increases breathing becomes difficult and noisy. There is usually a fever.

What are the treatment options?

Medical advice should be sought early, since severe breathing difficulties can occur rapidly. Treatment requires admission to hospital for intravenous antibiotics and fluids. If breathing difficulties are severe, a tube may need to be inserted through the mouth to help (intubation with an endotracheal tube), or tracheostomy (an incision into the upper air passage) may need to be performed.

What is the outlook?

The infection usually responds rapidly to treatment and within 48 hours most patients are making a good recovery. There are rarely any long-term consequences following epiglottitis.

EPISTAXIS

A complaint better known as a nosebleed.

What are the causes?

There is no obvious cause for around 85 per cent of nosebleeds, which are due to spontaneous rupture of a small blood vessel inside the nose. The remaining 15 per cent have a variety of causes, such as trauma to the nose (including picking!), infection, tumours, blood disorders, allergies and some medicines.

What are the treatment options?

First aid measures can be tried when a nosebleed starts (p.51). Where the blood vessel responsible can be seen at the front of the nose, cauterisation may be necessary for bleeds that do not settle. This is usually performed under a local anaesthetic to the inside of the nose and can be a little uncomfortable. A chemical stick or hot wire is used to seal the burst blood vessel.

If these remedies fail to stop the bleeding, the nose may need to be packed. This is a method of applying pressure to the bleeding spot by putting a dressing inside the nose. Various types of dressing are available. If the nose is packed, admission to hospital is usually necessary. Occasionally, the bleeding still fails to settle and then surgery is required to locate the bleeding vessel and deal with it under direct vision with the patient anaesthetised. Rarely, the main blood vessel in the neck, the carotid artery, may have to be tied to stop bleeding.

HEARING LOSS

Hearing loss, or deafness, affects a large number of people, and becomes more common as people age. The Medical Research Council (MRC) Institute of Hearing Research estimates that 1 in 5 people have hearing impairment that requires the use of a hearing aid.

What are the causes?

There are two types of hearing loss – sensorineural and conductive. Sensorineural hearing loss is when the inner ear is responsible for the deafness. The cochlea or the pathways from the cochlea to the brain are affected. The deafness may be present from birth, or may be acquired later in life. Some infections such as meningitis, measles and mumps can cause deafness, as can a skull fracture. The hearing loss of old age is sensorineural (p.146).

Conductive deafness is when sound cannot reach the inner ear (cochlea) due to disease or blockage in the middle ear or ear canal. Causes include wax, glue ear (p.144) and otosclerosis (p.145).

How is it diagnosed?

Hearing loss is measured by a hearing test called an audiogram (p.108). To distinguish between the two types of deafness, the test is performed using headphones and a bone vibrator placed behind the ear. If the hearing loss is conductive, the sounds will be heard better with the bone vibrator than the headphones.

What are the treatment options?

Sensorineural hearing loss can be helped by amplifying residual hearing with a hearing aid. Many types of hearing aid are available, both commercially and through the National Health Service. For the profoundly deaf, a cochlear implant may be offered after careful assessment. Conductive hearing loss is dealt with by treating the underlying cause where possible, for example grommet insertion for glue ear. Where treatment of the underlying condition is not possible or appropriate, a hearing aid can be worn with good effect.

What is the outlook?

To an extent this depends on the cause of the hearing loss, but hearing aid technology is improving all the time, with smaller and more sophisticated models coming onto the market. Many more profoundly deaf people are benefiting from cochlear implant surgery, and surgery for conductive hearing loss has been refined over the years. Screening of newborn babies for hearing ability can detect congenital hearing problems as soon as possible so that early treatment can be introduced to prevent delay in speech and language development.

Babies with hearing problems who receive hearing aids, visual and hearing stimulation, and who start learning to sign by the age of six months, are likely to develop good communication skills.

INFECTIOUS MONONUCLEOSIS

Commonly known as glandular fever, this is an infection caused by a virus.

What is the cause?

Glandular fever is caused by the Epstein-Barr virus. The virus is passed from person to person in saliva, which is why the illness is also known as the 'kissing disease'. It is most common in adolescents or young adults, but can occur in children and the middle aged.

What are the symptoms?

Some patients may be infected without showing any signs of illness. The classical symptoms, however, are:
- Sore throat, which may be severe enough to prevent swallowing of saliva, and occasionally difficulty in breathing may occur.
- Fever.
- Swelling of glands in the neck and sometimes elsewhere in the body.
- Lethargy and a general feeling of malaise.
- There may be some swelling around the eyes, and a rash may be present. (The rash may be part of the disease, but can also occur if a patient with glandular fever is prescribed the antibiotic ampicillin.)
- The liver and spleen may become enlarged and a small number of patients develop jaundice.

How is it diagnosed?

A blood test can show whether the symptoms are due to infectious mononucleosis.

What are the treatment options?

The viral infection must run its course, but symptoms can be relieved. The sore throat will respond to simple analgesics, such as paracetamol or ibuprofen, and these will also help with any fever. Plenty of fluids should be taken. If the patient cannot swallow fluids, they may need to be admitted to hospital for rehydration using a drip. Admission is also advised if there are breathing difficulties, and some patients may be given steroids while in hospital to treat this. It is usually advisable to avoid contact sports for a month or so if there has been enlargement of the spleen, in case it ruptures.

What is the outlook?

The infection usually lasts for 1 to 2 weeks but is often followed by some months of tiredness before complete recovery. Full activity should be encouraged as early as possible. About 1 in 2000 affected people develop a chronic or recurrent form that may last for several months.

LABYRINTHITIS

An inflammation of the inner ear leading to balance problems or dizziness.

What are the causes?

Infection of the inner ear is commonly due to a viral infection, but can occur following a bacterial infection of the middle ear (see Otitis media, p.144).

What are the symptoms?

- Viral labyrinthitis often starts with a viral illness: the patient feels unwell and has flu-like symptoms.
- This is followed by the onset of sudden severe dizziness associated with nausea and vomiting. The vertigo may be so severe that the patient can only lie still.

- The eyes dart rapidly from side to side; this is known as nystagmus (p.109).
- As the condition settles down, the dizziness starts to get better, but there may be residual feelings of unsteadiness when moving the head for some weeks or months.

How is it diagnosed?

Since this complaint is thought to be due to a viral infection, in most cases the diagnosis is made on history and examination. The ears are examined to ensure that there is no middle ear infection present to cause the inner ear inflammation, and if the history suggests a viral infection and the ears look healthy, no further investigation is required. If the dizziness does not seem to improve as expected – the condition usually resolves over days and weeks – other causes need to be looked for.

What are the treatment options?

With time, the brain starts to compensate for the dizziness, which gradually gets better. The worst of the illness is usually over within a few days, but residual

EXPERIENCING AN INNER EAR INFECTION

I had had a cold for a few days before the dizziness started. It came on suddenly out of the blue. The room started spinning and I couldn't focus – my eyes felt like they were jumping about. I thought I was going to faint and had to lie down. Then I felt sick and started to vomit.

My husband took me to an ENT clinic. After asking me how it had started and checking my ears, the doctor said it was probably a viral infection of the inner ear and gave me an injection to help the dizziness and sickness. I went home and lay down and within an hour I began to feel better. The sickness stopped and the dizziness was better as long as I lay still. The doctor, however, had urged me to get out of bed and move around as this would help my brain to start compensating for the upset to my balance, so I did this the next day. For some weeks, if I turned my head quickly the dizziness returned for a few minutes, but this slowly got better and after about six weeks I was back to normal.

unsteadiness and feelings of dizziness on certain movements can take weeks or even months to settle completely. During the worst of the infection, medication such as prochlorperazine can help to suppress any dizziness and feeling of nausea. Any residual imbalance or dizziness may be helped by exercises that encourage the brain to adapt to the changes caused by the infection in the inner ear. These are known as Cawthorne-Cooksey, or vestibular rehabilitation, exercises (p.76).

What is the outlook?

Nearly all cases resolve completely in time. If this does not happen, further investigation may be required to rule out other causes of balance problems such as Ménière's disease (p.140).

LARYNGITIS
Inflammation of the larynx, the part of the throat concerned with speaking.

What are the causes?
- Acute laryngitis is commonly caused by a viral infection or overuse of the voice, for example too much shouting at a football match.
- Chronic laryngitis is more likely to be associated with smoking, excess alcohol consumption, or long-term voice overuse by people such as lawyers, teachers and singers, or people who work in noisy environments, or even children who scream excessively.

What are the symptoms?
- Acute laryngitis may be associated with a viral upper respiratory tract infection, such as the common cold, with all the associated symptoms. The throat feels sore and the voice starts to become croaky or husky. If the voice is not rested at this stage it may disappear altogether for a while.
- Chronic laryngitis shares many of the symptoms of acute laryngitis, but often without pain.

How is it diagnosed?
Most cases of acute laryngitis get better very quickly without needing any treatment by a doctor. If seen by a doctor, the diagnosis is usually made on the history and, if necessary, by examining the larynx with a mirror or endoscope. The vocal cords will appear reddened and swollen, and other areas of the larynx may be inflamed.

Any hoarseness that does not resolve within 4–6 weeks needs further investigation to rule out cancer of the larynx (p.135), especially in high-risk groups such as smokers.

What are the treatment options?
- Acute laryngitis usually gets better without any specific treatment, since it is usually due to a viral infection or short-term voice abuse. Most cases respond to simple measures such as resting the voice, drinking plenty of fluids, steam inhalations and simple analgesia for the sore throat.
- Chronic laryngitis, once cancer has been ruled out, will usually get better if smoking ceases, and measures are taken as for acute laryngitis. If voice misuse is a contributory factor, speech therapy may be helpful. Occasionally, if the vocal cords have become very swollen, surgery may be helpful to reduce the swelling and so improve the voice.

LARYNGOMALACIA
A condition seen in newborn babies in which the tissues of the larynx are floppy, causing noisy breathing.

What are the causes?
The laryngeal tissues are floppy at birth due to immaturity of the supporting cartilage.

What are the symptoms?
The baby develops noisy or squeaky breathing, usually on breathing in, within an hour or two or up to several weeks after birth. The symptoms may be worsened by:
- feeding;
- lying on its back;
- infections such as colds;
- agitation.

Rarely, the condition may obstruct breathing.

How is it diagnosed?
If symptoms are mild and there is no interference with feeding, no further investigation is required, and the child merely needs checking at the clinic at regular intervals until it grows out of the condition.

If the symptoms are more severe or interfere with feeding, the larynx needs to be inspected: it is sometimes possible to do this in the ENT clinic with a very fine flexible endoscope if the baby is cooperative, but more usually a general anaesthetic is required.

What are the treatment options?
- Laryngomalacia gets better as the baby grows older and the cartilage supporting the larynx matures. For most children no treatment is necessary.
- If the condition is severe, it can interfere with feeding, since the baby finds it difficult to breathe and feed at the same time. The child may fail to gain weight and become undernourished. In such cases, and those where the breathing is severely affected, the larynx is usually examined under a general anaesthetic. This will confirm the diagnosis and make sure that there is no other reason for the problems encountered. At the same time, any surplus tissue that may be getting in the way of breathing can be removed. In very severe cases, where the baby is struggling to breathe adequately, a tracheostomy (p.129) may be necessary as a temporary measure until the condition starts to resolve.

What is the outlook?
The symptoms gradually improve with time. It can sometimes take a few years for the larynx to become firm enough to resist collapse on breathing in, but all children will grow out of the condition.

MENIERE'S DISEASE
First described in 1861 by Prosper Ménière, this condition of the inner ear is characterised by vertigo (dizziness), tinnitus and deafness.

What is the cause?
It is thought to be due to a sudden increase in the volume of fluid called endolymph in the inner ear. The cause of this increase is unknown, but is being actively researched. The condition is more common in middle age and appears to occur equally among women and men. There is often a history of migraine in the family, but the link is uncertain.

What are the symptoms?
The main feature of Ménière's disease is that it occurs in episodes, and in between sufferers are often well with few symptoms. The main symptoms are:
- **Dizziness (vertigo)** Attacks vary in frequency, with some patients having just one or two a year and others having more frequent episodes. The dizziness may last minutes or hours, with some patients experiencing nausea and vomiting during an attack. After an attack has finished, the sufferer may feel unwell for some days.

- **Tinnitus** A ringing or buzzing noise in the ear is often noticed during an attack. In the early stages of the disease, the tinnitus disappears completely between attacks, but as time goes by it can become constant.
- **Hearing loss** This is associated with the dizzy spells. At first it may be described as a feeling of fullness or blockage in the ear which gets better as the attack subsides, but as the attacks continue, the hearing recovers to a lesser degree after each attack, until a permanent sensorineural hearing loss (p.137) is experienced.

How is it diagnosed?

In the early stages there may be little to find, since all returns to normal between attacks. Patients are usually seen at an ENT clinic between attacks, and various tests are performed.

- **Hearing test** This is performed in all cases of suspected Ménière's disease and may show evidence of a sensorineural hearing loss. If the test is repeated at intervals between attacks, it may show the fluctuation of the hearing and eventually the gradually worsening and permanent hearing loss. Usually only one ear is affected, although about one-third of patients eventually go on to develop disease in the second ear.
- **Tests of vestibular function** These record the function of the part of the inner ear responsible for balance – this is the part responsible for the dizziness experienced by patients. A number of tests are available, including calorics and electrocochleography, or an MRI scan. It may sometimes be necessary to rule out the possibility of an acoustic neuroma (p.134) in a patient with hearing loss in one ear only, before assuming it is due to Ménière's disease.

What are the treatment options?

Treatment may be medical or surgical, and the simplest treatments are usually tried first.

Initially, most patients are treated medically. Lifestyle measures include stopping smoking, which will improve blood flow to the nerve endings of the inner ear; reducing the intake of salt to decrease the accumulation of fluid in the inner ear; and eliminating caffeine to avoid excess stimulation of the nerve endings. Patients are usually prescribed betahistine (marketed under the brandnames Serc, SERC or Betaserc) to increase blood flow in the inner ear. The drug helps to prevent attacks and is therefore taken on a long-term basis. Other drugs used to treat the attacks as they occur include prochlorperazine and cinnarizine; these will reduce the sickness associated with an attack, as well as alleviating the dizziness. Diuretics have also been tried, with varying success.

A procedure known as intratympanic gentamicin, in which an antibiotic called gentamicin is injected through the eardrum, can be carried out in an outpatient clinic. When used in doses to fight infection elsewhere in the body, this antibiotic can have the unfortunate side effect of damaging the inner ear, an effect that is exploited in this situation. The drug is put into the middle ear through the drum, with the intention of damaging that part of the inner ear responsible for balance and stopping the dizzy spells. The disadvantage of this treatment is that it can also destroy hearing in that ear. However, for those experiencing frequent severe attacks of dizziness that are very disabling, this may be a price worth paying.

Various techniques have been tried over the years to cure the condition by surgery. The simplest procedure is the insertion of a grommet (p.120). There is no good explanation as to why this should work – some have even claimed it is due to the placebo effect – but in some patients the procedure brings relief of symptoms.

The main surgical treatment for Ménière's disease is endolymphatic saccus decompression. The sac is part of the inner ear and is normally covered by the bone of the skull. By opening up the area behind the ear (known as the mastoid bone) the saccus is exposed, and it is thought this enables it to expand freely when the fluid in the inner ear increases during an attack.

A more radical operation is one that cuts the nerve running from the balance apparatus to the brain. This requires the skull to be opened and hence carries more risk of complications, but does appear to relieve symptoms. If there is little useful hearing left in the affected ear, a labyrinthectomy may be carried out to cure the symptoms, but this will destroy both the inner ear and any hearing.

What is the outlook?

In many cases, the disease seems to burn itself out after a number of years. The dizzy attacks cease and the hearing stops deteriorating, although it does not recover. The tinnitus may also remain. Prior to reaching this stage, many cases are well controlled by medication. Research continues into this distressing condition.

Some 90 per cent of patients report relief of symptoms of Ménière's disease after endolymphatic saccus decompression, but only 60 per cent claim continued relief after five years.

MOTION SICKNESS
A feeling of nausea that may lead to actual vomiting, usually experienced while travelling.

What are the causes?
The balance part of the inner ear is very sensitive to changes in position. In some people it is so sensitive that even minor frequent changes, such as that experienced when travelling in a car, is enough to confuse the brain. So many different signals are received in rapid succession that the brain can no longer tell which way up the body is or which way it is facing. This leads to the stimulation of various receptors which in turn leads to feelings of sickness and can in extremes cause vomiting.

What are the treatment options?
Various medications are available for motion sickness. Some, such as hyoscine, prevent the onset of symptoms if taken in advance of travel. Antihistamines such as cinnarizine, also taken before travelling, can help to stave off sickness and have fewer side effects, but they are a little less effective. These drugs all work by suppressing the balance mechanism of the inner ear and the part of the brain responsible for vomiting.

HELP YOUR DOCTOR TO HELP YOU

Describing ENT symptoms

When describing symptoms, it will help your doctor to help you if you can be precise about them. A clear history will enable the doctor to make a final diagnosis and prescribe appropriate medication. Note such factors as:

• *Does dizziness feel like the room spinning or just a light-headed feeling? Does it happen only with certain movements of the head or can it come on even when sitting still?*

• *Does motion sickness come on with every journey; only on certain forms of transport; or at other times, such as in the cinema?*

• *Are nosebleeds common, infrequent, only happen after a cold or other infection?*

• *Is snoring an every-night occurrence or does it only happen after drinking alcohol late?*

What is the outlook?
Adaptation does occur in people who are in a prolonged situation that induces motion sickness, such as on a ship. Many young sailors suffer from sickness on a first long sea voyage, but for most the sickness gradually settles until they have no further problems.

NASAL POLYPOSIS
A condition in which the membrane lining the nasal cavity becomes thickened and produces swellings.

When the lining of the nose becomes inflamed it becomes swollen. If this swelling continues untreated, the lining becomes more and more swollen and areas fill with fluid. These gelatinous sacs on the nasal or sinus lining are called polyps (a swelling with a stalk).

What are the causes?
The initial inflammation may be triggered by a number of factors including chronic infection and allergy. There are certain groups of patients, such as asthmatics, in whom polyps are more likely to form, particularly if they are allergic to aspirin.

What are the symptoms?
While they are small, the polyps may not show any symptoms, although if associated with allergies the symptoms may initially be put down to these. The most common complaints are of nasal obstruction and nasal speech. As the polyps enlarge, there may be a clear watery discharge from the nose. The sense of smell is often poor, and this affects the sense of taste. There is sometimes headache and pressure across the face, and sinusitis may occur. If ignored for a long time, the polyps can become so large that they hang out of the nose and cause it to widen.

How is it diagnosed?
It is easy to see even small polyps using an endoscope. If surgery is necessary, a **CT** scan is sometimes performed to help plan the procedure, or if there are polyps in only one side of the nose, to rule out tumour. Other tests relate to the underlying causes, such as skin testing for allergies.

What are the treatment options?
Unless the polyps are very large, the first choice for the majority of cases is medical treatment. This consists of sprays or drops into the nose which contain a small dose

of steroid that acts on the polyps directly to reduce the inflammation and cause them to shrink. Very little of the steroid administered in this way is absorbed into the body, so the usual side effects associated with steroid use are rarely encountered. Occasionally, a short course of steroid tablets may be used to get things under control.

Surgery is appropriate in those cases where the polyps are large or if sinusitis (p.150) is an associated problem. Most surgery is performed using an endoscope, but other types of surgery are occasionally used to treat severe cases. After surgery most patients need medical treatment to help prevent recurrence of the polyps.

What is the outlook?
For a proportion of patients, particularly those with asthma or aspirin allergy, the polyps will keep coming back. It is thought that prolonged treatment with drops or sprays helps to increase the time between recurrences, but it may not prevent them completely. Nasal polyposis is an area of much ongoing research, and the pathways involved in inflammation are constantly being looked at to develop new drugs that may suppress the underlying background of inflammation in patients with polyps.

Ongoing research into drugs to combat nasal polyps may mean that one day most patients will be treated solely with drugs and surgery becomes a rarity.

OBSTRUCTIVE SLEEP APNOEA
A condition where breathing is obstructed during sleep to the extent that breathing stops and the sufferer wakes.

Obstructive sleep apnoea can affect adults and children. It is more common in adult males than females, and affects younger children rather than older.

What are the causes?
In adults the airway becomes obstructed during sleep by collapse of the soft tissues from the nose to the voice box. In children obstruction is usually due to the relatively large size of the adenoids and tonsils. As the person breathes in, the tissues cause complete obstruction of the airway, and no air is actually drawn in. In adults, certain factors make sleep apnoea more likely. These include:
• obesity;
• alcohol consumption;
• age – the condition is more common as age increases;
• sex – it is more common in males.

What are the symptoms?
The patient's history is very important, in particular that from the sleeping partner or parent. It can be very frightening for the onlooker to see a person struggling for breath and many report waking the sufferer at intervals to make them breathe. If left alone, the affected person will breathe spontaneously as their level of consciousness rises due to the lowered oxygen levels and increased carbon dioxide in the blood. The resulting interrupted sleep can lead to a number of symptoms during the day.
• **Daytime sleepiness** This may be responsible for a number of road accidents as people fall asleep while driving. Children may be miserable during the day and need more naps than usual.
• **Morning headaches** These may be due to the raised levels of carbon dioxide in the blood and lack of oxygen.
• **Lack of concentration.**
• **Impotence.**

How is it diagnosed?
To make a diagnosis a sleep study must be undertaken. The subject is attached to monitors while sleeping. These record, among other things, periods of obstruction when no air passes, the levels of oxygen in the blood, blood pressure and heart rate. Admission to hospital overnight is usual. Some specialists perform a sleep nasendoscopy, giving the patient a drug to induce sleep and inserting an endoscope through the nose to examine the entire larynx.

How is it treated?
Simple measures such as losing weight and reducing alcohol consumption are recommended for all adults. For severe sleep apnoea CPAP (continuous positive airway pressure) is the treatment of choice. This involves wearing a mask at night that provides air at a pressure that keeps the airway open. In children, the removal of the adenoids and tonsils is recommended. Less severe OSA may be managed by a mandibular advancement splint – a type of gum shield worn at night that opens the airway.

OTITIS EXTERNA
Infection or inflammation of the ear canal.

What are the causes?
Otitis externa may be acute or chronic. The chronic cases tend to be associated with skin problems, such as eczema, which predisposes the skin of the ear canal to infection,

particularly when wet. Acute infections are often secondary to other factors, such as trauma to the ear canal by the use of cotton buds or fingernails for cleaning the ear, or water in the ear when swimming or bathing. The infection may be bacterial or sometimes fungal.

What are the symptoms?
Symptoms include pain, swelling of the ear canal or whole ear, discharge from the ear and itching.

How is it diagnosed?
Otitis externa is diagnosed on patient history and examination. In the event of no response to the prescribed treatment, a swab may be taken from the ear canal to see which micro-organisms are responsible for the infection.

How is it treated?
Discharge in the ear canal should be cleaned prior to using any drops. If the ear canal is swollen a dressing in the canal may be required, since drops may not reach the deeper parts of the canal. Ear drops containing antibiotics and steroids to reduce the swelling are usually prescribed.

In severe cases with spread of infection to the whole ear or face, admission to hospital for intravenous antibiotics may be advised. For chronic eczema of the ear canal, steroid ear drops and creams may be recommended. In all cases it is important to keep water out of the ears. Generally, cleaning the ears with cotton buds or any other implement is not recommended.

OTITIS MEDIA
An inflammation of the middle ear.

The middle ear is the space behind the eardrum, which can become inflamed during an infection.

What are the causes?
Otitis media may be acute or chronic. Acute otitis media is often associated with upper respiratory tract infections. It is caused by infection of the middle ear as bacteria reach the middle ear through the eustachian tube. It is more common in young children. Most children have frequent colds, and the adenoids may be enlarged, causing blockage of the eustachian tube.

Chronic otitis media, or otitis media with effusion, is also known as glue ear. The fundamental problem here is eustachian tube dysfunction. The pressure behind the eardrum is unable to equalise, as air cannot get up the tube. Consequently, the pressure in the middle ear falls. This causes inflammation of the middle ear lining and fluid is produced which fills the middle ear space. The eustachian tube may be functioning poorly because of adenoidal hypertrophy, immaturity, problems such as cleft palate and tumour in the back of the nose.

What are the symptoms?
Acute otitis media causes pain, fever and deafness. If untreated, the eardrum may burst: this relieves the pain, but the fluid then leaks from the ear. Chronic otitis media, or glue ear, is usually characterised by hearing loss. Because the fluid has built up gradually, it is usually painless unless infected.

How is it diagnosed?
Examination of the ear reveals the presence of fluid behind the eardrum, and a hearing test confirms a conductive hearing loss. If the eardrum is not moving due to fluid behind it, the tympanometry test (p.108) will produce a flat trace.

What are the treatment options?
Acute otitis media will often get better within 24 hours without treatment. If not, it responds well to antibiotics. These will usually be taken orally, but if it is felt that the infection has spread into the mastoid bone, a condition known as mastoiditis, intravenous antibiotics are

Why do some children with glue ear have their adenoids removed?

The adenoids are lumps of lymphoid tissue found at the back of the nose, which are similar to the tonsils. They tend to be biggest between the ages of three and eight and then shrink in size. Because of their position at the back of the nose it is thought that they can cause blockage of the eustachian tube and therefore play a role in the formation of glue ear and acute otitis media. There is still much debate as to whether removal has much effect on the control of otitis media, however. Some studies show a significant improvement, especially in older children.

ASK THE EXPERT

required. Chronic otitis media, or glue ear, is often a self-limiting condition, especially in children. There is, therefore, a good case for watching and waiting. Most specialists recommend review after three months, since a proportion of children get better without treatment during that period.

Further treatment is usually recommended in the following situations:

- Persistent deafness causing behavioural problems or difficulties at school.
- Where the eardrum is becoming unhealthy and is in danger of collapsing. This can be a precursor to the formation of a benign tumour of the middle ear known as a cholesteatoma.

For chronic otitis media, the usual treatment is the insertion of a grommet, or ventilation tube. The adenoids may sometimes be removed.

If the main problem is hearing loss and the parents are against surgical intervention, a hearing aid can be useful. In adults with glue ear on one side only, tests should be done to exclude a tumour at the back of the nose when the grommet is inserted.

What is the outlook?

The natural history of both acute and chronic otitis media is one of spontaneous improvement. Most children will grow out of the problem, so intervention depends upon the severity of the symptoms. If grommets are inserted, they usually expel themselves after about a year, and only one-quarter of children will need another set.

OTOSCLEROSIS

The formation of new bone in the middle ear which interferes with the conduction of sound to the cochlea.

Otosclerosis is an inherited disease in which abnormal bone grows in the middle ear. This results in deafness because the small bones of the middle ear (ossicles) become fixed and so are unable to conduct sound from the ear drum to the inner ear efficiently. Occasionally, the inner ear is also involved.

What are the symptoms?

Deafness is the primary symptom and tends to occur before the age of 30. It particularly affects women. Many patients also suffer with tinnitus (p.152), especially if the inner ear is involved.

How is it diagnosed?

A hearing test typically shows a marked deafness due to poor conduction of sound from the outside world to the inner ear. If the inner ear is involved, there is an additional sensory element to the hearing loss.

What are the treatment options?

Some people with mild otosclerosis do not require treatment. However, in those with significant deafness, the two main options are a hearing aid or surgery. A hearing aid is simple, effective and risk free but has the obvious disadvantage of being visible behind and within the ear. The operation – called a stapedectomy – involves drilling a tiny 0.6mm wide hole in the stapes and bypassing the fixed segment by inserting a piston. The operation is successful in more than 90 per cent of cases but certain risks are associated with it. In particular, there is a 1 per cent chance of losing the hearing in that ear. Some patients suffer with vertigo, but this settles after a few days.

Up to 10 per cent of the population is thought to be affected by otosclerosis to some degree, although only 1 per cent notices any significant hearing loss. Most affected people have the disease in both ears.

PHARYNGITIS

Inflammation of the lining of either the throat or the pharynx.

Pharyngitis is very common and may be acute or chronic. The acute form is probably the commonest cause of 'sore throat' in adults.

What are the causes?

Acute pharyngitis is most commonly caused by a viral infection but it can be bacterial in origin. In contrast, the chronic form of the disease may be due to irritation by cigarette smoke or alcohol. It may also follow contact with infected mucous in a patient with sinusitis, or be due to acid reflux from the stomach. In many patients no cause can be identified. A chronic sore throat may be a symptom of malignancy, so a sore throat that lasts more than four weeks should be seen by an ENT specialist.

What are the symptoms?

Both acute and chronic pharyngitis are characterised by a sore throat. In addition, acute pharyngitis is often associated with a multitude of other symptoms depending on which other areas are affected. There is often a fever, with general malaise, and there may be a runny or blocked nose, hoarseness if the larynx is affected or cough if the lungs are affected. In contrast, chronic pharyngitis often has no symptoms except sore throat. However, there may be symptoms of the underlying condition, for example of sinusitis or of gastro-oesophageal reflux.

How is it diagnosed?
The symptoms are the most important aid to diagnosis, but examination may show an inflamed pharynx with infected mucous present. The examination may not show anything specific in those with chronic pharyngitis.

What are the treatment options?
Acute pharyngitis is self-limiting and usually settles after 4 to 5 days. Treatment involves pain relief and plenty of fluids. Antibiotics are rarely required, since the underlying cause is usually viral. Treatment of chronic pharyngitis depends on the underlying cause. If smoking or alcohol consumption are contributing factors, they should be stopped. Sinusitis or gastro-oesophageal reflux are treated as appropriate. Examination of the pharynx, under anaesthetic if necessary, should be carried out in selected cases to make sure there is not an underlying malignancy.

HELP YOUR DOCTOR TO HELP YOU

Describing a sore throat
Your doctor needs to know the following factors about a sore throat in order to reach a diagnosis and recommend appropriate treatment.

- *How long the sore throat has persisted, whether you have had a sore throat before, and whether family members also have sore throats, or have had them recently.*

- *Whether the pain is worse at night or in the morning, or if it prevents you from sleeping.*

- *Does anything relieve it (such as a warm drink or painkillers) or make it worse (such as swallowing or breathing through the mouth)?*

- *Whether your voice is affected: has it almost gone or is it simply hoarse?*

- *Is the sore throat getting better or worse, or is it about the same?*

PRESBYACUSIS
Age-related hearing loss.

It is an inevitability that our hearing deteriorates as we get older. This can cause considerable functional impairment in the elderly person, who may also have other medical problems to contend with.

What is the cause?
The cause of presbyacusis is not known but the condition involves a deterioration in the number of nerve fibres supplying the cochlea and in the hair cells responsible for detecting sound. Thus the quality of the information passing to the brain from the inner ear deteriorates.

What are the symptoms?
Deterioration of hearing in both ears is the primary symptom. A loss of the ability to discriminate between words makes understanding speech a problem, especially in noisy environments. There may also be distortion of sounds. The ear looks normal when examined.

How is it diagnosed?
A hearing test confirms the diagnosis in conjunction with a thorough medical history. There is, typically, a particular loss of hearing in the high frequencies.

What are the treatment options?
Early presbyacusis may not require any treatment except reassurance that there is no underlying problem with the ears. As the process progresses and the hearing loss becomes severe, the best method of treatment is a hearing aid. There is no surgical method of improving the hearing of people with this condition.

What is the outlook?
The deterioration is often progressive and eventually those who are worst affected can become profoundly deaf. There is a wide spectrum of severity, however, and many people only experience mild degrees of presbyacusis.

QUINSY
An abscess next to the tonsil following acute tonsillitis.

Tonsillar infection is very common and in the most severe cases can result in the formation of pus and the development of an abscess in the tissues around the tonsil, hence its alternative name of peritonsillar abscess. This often makes the symptoms much more severe. It tends to affect young adults, and is rare in children.

What are the causes?
The cause is the same as that for tonsillitis: an acute bacterial infection. The reason why some people should develop an abscess while others do not is not understood.

What are the symptoms?
Sore throat, difficulty swallowing and fever are present, as they are for tonsillitis. However, the pain may be more severe, particularly on the affected side. It may be difficult to open the mouth since the abscess causes inflammation of the muscles involved in opening the mouth and there is often a 'plummy' quality to the voice due to the swelling in the throat. If it is not treated, the swelling can affect breathing and can therefore be life-threatening.

How is it diagnosed?
The typical appearance of the throat is of a striking swelling in the area just above the upper part of the affected tonsil. The presence of pus when the abscess is opened confirms the diagnosis.

What are the treatment options?
Pain relief and antibiotics are an important part of treating this problem. However, like any abscess, it will rarely resolve while there is still a collection of pus present. Thus, the abscess must be drained. Traditionally, after anaesthetising the area, the abscess was incised using a knife. More recently ENT surgeons have favoured removing the pus using a needle and syringe. This is often less painful and less traumatic to the lining of the throat.

What is the outlook?
The peritonsillar infection usually resolves quickly once the abscess is drained. Those who experience more than one episode of quinsy are usually advised to undergo tonsillectomy in order to prevent further problems.

RHINITIS
Inflammation of the membranes lining the nose.

Rhinitis is a very common condition that affects 1 in 6 people and its incidence is increasing. The lining of the nose is continuous with that of the sinuses and inflammation in the nose goes hand in hand with inflammation of the sinuses. Rhinitis is also frequently associated with asthma.

What are the causes?
Rhinitis may be part of a viral upper respiratory tract infection – 'the common cold' – or it may be secondary to a bacterial infection as with acute sinusitis. There is also evidence that reactions to fungus may be responsible for some cases of rhinitis. Other forms of the disease are due to allergy and there are many possible allergens. The most common is pollen and this constitutes 'hayfever'. Other common allergens include dust, dust mites, feathers and animal fur. The inflammation may also be part of a more generalised disease such as cystic fibrosis or rheumatoid arthritis. In some people there is no obvious cause.

What are the symptoms?
People suffering with this condition may experience a number of symptoms. There may be nasal blockage, runny nose, mucous dripping down the back of the nose, sneezing or nasal itching. Secondary symptoms such as facial pain and loss of the sense of smell may also occur.

How is it diagnosed?
The diagnosis is based on the symptoms and confirmed by clinical examination. The lining of the nose typically looks swollen and inflamed and there is usually mucous within the nose which may be watery in the case of allergy-induced rhinitis or green in the case of bacterial infection. Skin prick allergy tests confirm whether or not there is an allergic element.

A number of more specialised tests are available to help diagnose some of the rarer causes of the disease, and in those people who do not respond to treatment a CT scan of the sinuses may be required.

What are the treatment options?
This depends on the cause of the problem. For those with allergic rhinitis, one of the most important aspects of treatment is advice on avoiding the allergen that is causing it. Because there is no cure for this condition, the other arm of treatment is symptomatic relief. Several effective medications are available, the mainstay of treatment being topical steroid nasal sprays or drops. These generally have very low absorption rates and are, therefore, rarely associated with side effects, although dryness and occasional nosebleeds can occur.

In those with severe and resistant symptoms a course of oral steroids can be taken. For those people suffering with sneezing, itching or runny nose, oral anti-histamines can be used. There is also a topical preparation available for external use. Decongestants can be used temporarily but tend to make the symptoms worse if used over a prolonged period.

Rhinitis is the most common chronic illness of human beings.

What is the outlook?

There is no cure for most forms of rhinitis but in most cases the symptoms can be effectively controlled with the right advice and medication. Those who have persistent problems despite these measures may benefit from investigation of their sinuses. This is carried out by a telescopic technique and if necessary by CT scanning.

RUPTURED EAR DRUM
A hole that develops in the ear drum.

Rupture, or perforation, of the ear drum can occur as a result of middle ear infection, injury or following surgery on the ear. Repeated grommet insertion (p.120) can result in persistent perforation. In most cases the ear drum heals completely, but occasionally the process is incomplete and the individual is left with a hole in the drum.

What are the symptoms?

If the perforation is traumatic, there will be pain, deafness and often a bloody discharge from the ear. If there is injury to the inner ear as well, in a skull fracture for example, there may be dizziness and deafness. If the rupture is the result of infection, the symptoms will include fever and general malaise, together with deafness and a yellow or green discharge from the ear. Once the acute event is over, there may be no symptoms. In fact, some people will have a perforated ear drum and not even be aware of it. In those who do have symptoms, the most common are deafness and recurrent infections, particularly after swimming or bathing in contaminated water.

How is it diagnosed?

The diagnosis is made by examining the ear. The hole is usually clearly visible and the structures of the middle ear can often be seen, too. Tests of the functioning of the middle ear (tympanometry, p.108) can also be used to confirm the diagnosis.

SUFFERING A RUPTURED EAR DRUM

I've been diving for several years now and I rarely have any problems with my ears. Last summer, though, on a diving holiday, I mistimed my ascent and ended up rupturing my right ear drum. It was really painful at first, then after a few hours it just ached. I also had some bleeding from the ear.

More worrying than these symptoms, however, was the hearing loss. I went deaf and developed a ringing in my ear. The local doctor confirmed that I'd ruptured the ear drum and banned me from diving until I'd had the ear checked by a specialist.

Over the next few days the pain settled down and the ringing went away, much to my relief. My hearing also came back, and by the time I got back home and saw the specialist the hole had healed up. The specialist explained that most ruptures heal by themselves. I'm glad I didn't need surgery, and will take even more care with my dives in future.

What are the treatment options?

Infection in the middle ear should be treated with oral or local antibiotics, although there is some concern that certain local antibiotics can damage the cochlea, resulting in further deafness. Traumatic perforations usually heal by themselves after two or three weeks, so a doctor will simply observe the drum during that time.

If a perforation is persistent, a number of options are available. No treatment is needed if the perforation is not causing problems, although patients are advised to keep the ear dry to avoid infection. If the only symptom is hearing loss, this can be overcome with a hearing aid. If there is recurrent infection, or significant hearing loss and the patient does not wish to have a hearing aid, surgical repair can be carried out. The basic principle is to cover the perforation with tissue from elsewhere in the body, often from the temple of the face. This acts as a scaffolding so that the remaining drum can heal and fill in the defect. The operation is successful in around 80 per cent of cases.

SINGER'S NODES
Swellings or nodules which develop on the vocal cords as a result of poor voice habits.

Singer's nodes or nodules are a common complaint and can occur in both children and adults. They tend to affect women more than men. They are formed as a result of overuse or misuse of the voice. Thus, those who sing, talk a lot or frequently shout are most likely to develop a problem. A portion of each side of the vocal cord becomes swollen because of the trauma and, if the misuse continues, the swollen area becomes scarred. Once this stage is reached, the damage is often irreversible.

What are the symptoms?
The voice becomes breathy, husky and low pitched because the two sides of the vocal cords are no longer able to vibrate and come together effectively.

How is it diagnosed?
The definitive diagnosis is made by examining the voice box with a flexible endoscope. This allows identification of the nodules and exclusion of any other disease, such as a vocal cord paralysis or a malignancy. A more detailed examination of vocal cord function can be obtained using a special endoscope attached to a video that allows a real-time recording of vocal cord movements.

Are nodules on the vocal cords an early sign of throat cancer?

No – nodules are benign. They develop as a result of overuse or abuse of the voice and cause the vocal cords to swell and harden, which eventually results in hoarseness. Since hoarseness is also one of the symptoms of throat cancer, an ENT specialist will take a biopsy of any nodules to ensure that they are benign, but there is usually no cause for concern. Nodules respond best to voice rest and speech therapy to ensure that the poor habits that caused them are not continued. Some surgeons do opt to remove nodules, but the available evidence suggests that, without speech therapy to train a patient to use the voice wisely, nodules are likely to return.

ASK THE EXPERT

What are the treatment options?
The main aim of treatment is to re-educate the voice and correct the bad habits that have led to the formation of nodules. Exercises are recommended to reduce stress on the voice, eliminate the damaging habits and teach the individual how to use the voice correctly. The majority of vocal nodules will resolve in this way. Complete voice rest can also be successful, but it is difficult to maintain for an adequate length of time and does not correct the underlying problem, so the nodules tend to recur once the patient starts using the voice again. Close examination of the voice box under a general anaesthetic and removal the nodules by microsurgery is sometimes necessary.

SINUSITIS
Inflammation of the sinuses.

In the majority of cases inflammation of the sinuses goes hand in hand with inflammation of the nose. Hence a more correct term for this disease is rhinosinusitis.

What are the causes?
As with rhinitis, there are many different causes. It may be allergic in origin or infective. Infection may be viral, as with the common cold, or bacterial. There is increasing evidence for a fungal cause in some cases. Any infection can be acute or chronic. Similarly, it may be secondary to a more generalised illness, such as cystic fibrosis, rheumatoid arthritis or Wegener's granulomatosis.

What are the symptoms?
This depends on the cause, but typical symptoms are nasal blockage and runny nose, which may be watery in allergic causes, or thick and yellow or green in cases of infection. There is often mucous dripping into the throat from the back of the nose and facial pain due to pressure build-up in the sinuses. There may also be a loss of smell.

In severe infective cases, complications can develop. These include infection around the eye that can potentially damage vision, infection of the bone forming the walls of the sinuses, and spread of the infection to the brain or its coverings, resulting in meningitis or brain abscess.

How is it diagnosed?
The diagnosis is made on the patient's description of the symptoms and then confirmed by physical examination. The nasal lining is swollen and inflamed and there is a

discharge within the nose. In difficult cases, those which fail to respond to treatment or are suspected of having complications, a CT scan of the sinuses is carried out.

What are the treatment options?

The treatment depends on the underlying cause. Chronic inflammation due to allergy should be treated in the same way as allergic rhinitis (p.147) and includes avoiding allergens, and using steroids inside the nose and anti-histamines. Bacterial rhinosinusitis is treated with oral antibiotics, together with a short course of a decongestant followed by a steroid applied inside the nose. Viral rhinosinusitis requires only treatment of symptoms. Fungal sinusitis may require anti-fungal medications. If medical treatment fails, surgical drainage of the sinuses can be carried out, usually by endoscopic techniques.

What is the outlook?

Infective sinusitis can resolve completely with treatment. There is no cure for allergic rhinosinusitis, but in most patients good symptomatic relief can be obtained.

SNORING

Noise generated during sleep due to partial obstruction of the upper airway.

The number of people who snore has probably risen over the past few decades as a result of an increase in the number of people who are overweight, perhaps the most common contributing factor. However, the number of people consulting their doctor and ENT specialists for the problem has risen even faster, which partly reflects increased awareness of the availability of treatments. Snoring itself often causes significant disturbance, particularly to partners. In a proportion of cases it is associated with intermittent complete obstruction of the airway – obstructive sleep apnoea, or OSA (p.143).

What are the causes?

The noise of snoring occurs as a result of vibrations that develop between the soft palate or the walls of the pharynx. These are particularly likely to develop if the airway is narrowed for some reason. In adults, sites of narrowing include the nose, due to deviation of the nasal septum or rhinitis, and the throat, due to a floppy soft palate, bulky tongue or generalised narrowing of the pharynx as a result of obesity. Alcohol abuse also

predisposes people to snoring and OSA. In children, the adenoids and tonsils are proportionally larger than they are in adults. They can, therefore, cause narrowing of the airway and thus snoring and obstructive sleep apnoea.

What are the symptoms?

Simple snorers usually have no other symptoms except snoring. It is their partners who suffer with lack of sleep, leading to tiredness, irritability and loss of concentration the following day. The partner often resorts to sleeping in a separate room if possible, and in the most extreme cases marital difficulties can arise. It is important to have the partner present when discussing the problem. In contrast, those suffering with obstructive sleep apnoea suffer themselves from daytime tiredness, poor concentration, personality change and increased risk of road traffic accidents. The low oxygen levels in the blood that result from OSA can cause high blood pressure, excessive strain on the heart and an irregular heartbeat.

How is it diagnosed?

The most important aspects of diagnosis are to identify whether or not the snorer suffers with obstructive sleep apnoea and the site from which the obstruction originates. A combination of the symptoms that the person describes and thorough clinical examination usually answers these questions. The nose and throat are examined with a flexible telescope, and the patient's sleep patterns are assessed formally in an overnight sleep study.

Are all snorers at risk of obstructive sleep apnoea?

Snoring is a very common problem that in itself causes more difficulties for the partner than it does for the snorer. It results from the vibration of two adjacent surfaces in the lining of the nose or throat and is more likely to occur if these structures are narrowed for some reason, for example, as a result of obesity. In more extreme cases, the throat can become temporarily blocked during sleep resulting in sleep apnoea. Not everyone who snores suffers with sleep apnoea, but many snorers are at risk of developing the problem, especially those who are overweight and make no attempt to control this.

ASK THE EXPERT

Laser-assisted uvulopalatoplasty

Developed in France in the early 1990s, laser-assisted uvulopalatoplasty is carried out to reduce snoring and sleep apnoea. The technique involves the removal by laser of part of the uvula and back of the soft palate to widen the airway. Usually only one session of treatment is needed. The laser cuts down on bleeding and on post-operative pain, but studies suggest mixed results. Some document improvements in snoring in up to 80 per cent of patients. The success rate depends on correct evaluation to identify only palatal snorers.

What are the treatment options?

People with a simple snoring problem do not necessarily require any medical treatment. Reassurance that there is no serious underlying pathological cause, together with appropriate weight loss and reduction of alcohol consumption are often all that is required. If the nose is responsible for the obstruction, any septal deviation can be surgically corrected and any rhinitis can be treated. If the problem arises from the soft palate, surgical shortening of the uvula or stiffening of the palate by excision of excess tissue can be carried out.

A bulky tongue base can be dealt with using a special splint at night – a plastic device similar to orthodontic braces – to bring the jaw forward and increase the volume of the airway. If the obstruction originates from the throat, the airways can be kept open overnight by increasing the pressure inside the throat using a special mask (continuous positive airway pressure). This is often effective, but many people find the mask uncomfortable. In the most extreme cases of obstructive sleep apnoea a tracheostomy (p.129) can be life-saving. In children, an adenoidectomy or tonsillectomy is usually successful in resolving the problem.

STRIDOR

Noisy breathing, resulting from partial obstruction of the airway at or below the level of the voice box.

Stridor is often confused with the wheeze that is symptomatic of asthma. The main difference between them, however, is that stridor tends to be a difficulty with breathing in, whereas the wheeze from asthma tends to be a difficulty with breathing out. A third condition, stertor, is noisy breathing due to partial obstruction of the airway above the larynx, for example by large tonsils.

What are the causes?

The causes of stridor can be divided into problems that the individual was born with (congenital) and those that are acquired through some event or disease process. Congenital problems include:

- weakness of the structure of the voice box or trachea, which results in collapse;
- laryngotracheomalacia – congenital narrowing of the voice box or trachea (stenosis);
- benign tumours of the airway such as haemangiomata.

Acquired causes include:

- injury from thermal or chemical burns or direct trauma;
- inflammation as a result of infection or other inflammatory condition;
- inhaled foreign bodies within the airway;
- paralysis of one or both of the vocal cords;
- swelling within the airway following an allergic reaction;
- narrowing of the airway due to a tumour.

What are the symptoms?

Noisy breathing, together with difficulty in breathing in, are features of stridor. In severe cases, inadequate oxygen levels in the blood can make the situation life-threatening. Other symptoms depend on the underlying cause. For example, an infection in the voice box may cause a high temperature and a hoarse voice. Any tumour affecting the voice box causes hoarseness, and – if it is malignant – there may be difficulty in swallowing and weight loss.

How is it diagnosed?

The condition is easily diagnosed by listening to the character of the person's breathing. Examination of the voice box with a flexible telescope identifies the underlying cause. It may be necessary to examine the voice box under a general anaesthetic to assess the situation more accurately, especially in children. If a specific lesion is identified, it can be easily biopsied while the individual is anaesthetised.

What are the treatment options?

This depends on the underlying cause. Children with laryngomalacia (p.140) can often be treated before any real problems arise and the excess floppy tissue removed under anaesthetic. In cases of stenosis of the voice box, it is possible to widen the narrow portion surgically; it may be necessary to carry out a tracheostomy (p.129) in the interim. Traumatic injury to the voice box often requires surgical intervention, which may also involve a tracheostomy in the first instance. Infection is treated with antibiotics and in the majority of cases no further treatment is required. Foreign bodies can be removed safely under a brief general anaesthetic.

Treatment of tumours in the larynx involves removal of the lesion. Benign tumours can often be removed through the mouth. Traditionally, once a malignant tumour was large enough to cause stridor, removal involved a partial or total laryngectomy (removal of the voice box). More recently, removal of cancerous tumours has been carried out successfully through the mouth, using a special laser.

TINNITUS
The sensation of hearing a sound in the absence of any external noise.

Tinnitus is a very common problem, particularly among the elderly. In severe cases it can become quite disabling.

What is the cause?
Virtually any disease of the external, middle or inner ear can cause tinnitus. For example, tinnitus occurs with impacted wax, noise-induced hearing loss, Ménière's disease, and rarely tumours of the auditory nerve (see Acoustic neuroma, p.134, and Otosclerosis, p.145). It is also associated with a number of conditions including anaemia, high blood pressure and neurological diseases such as multiple sclerosis, and it can be provoked by medication, including aspirin and some antibiotics.

However, most people who suffer with tinnitus do not have any associated ear disease and in these cases the underlying cause is not known. Among the theories put forward to explain the problem is that it may be due to increased or decreased activity in the auditory nerve, or to cross-stimulation of adjacent nerve fibres within the auditory nerve. Alternatively, it may be due to abnormal function of the central processing of auditory information.

What are the symptoms?
Tinnitus can be intermittent or continuous and its character varies from person to person: it may be heard as a buzzing, humming or whooshing, among other

Is there a cure for tinnitus?

There is no cure for tinnitus, but some support groups advocate the four Rs as a means of living with and overcoming the condition.

- RECOGNITION A doctor can determine that there is no underlying illness and reassure a patient that the condition is not life threatening and that strategies exist to overcome it.
- RELAXATION Relaxing the body breaks the vicious cycle of tinnitus – worry – tension – tinnitus seems worse – more worry, and so on.
- RETRAINING A sufferer can train the mind to become used to tinnitus by listening to other sounds. Taped music, played at just below the level of the tinnitus, for several hours a day, often helps a patient to 'tune out' the tinnitus.
- RECREATION Keeping physically and mentally active may make tinnitus recede into the background so a sufferer is not conscious of it for long periods of the day.

ASK THE EXPERT

noises. It is usually most noticeable in a quiet environment, especially at night. Tinnitus typically affects both ears, but a single ear can be affected and in this instance it is important to rule out an underlying cause such as an acoustic neuroma. In most tinnitus patients the clinical examination is entirely normal. However, the majority have some degree of hearing loss, as confirmed by a hearing test. It is important to find out what sort of impact the tinnitus is having on the individual's life, since this will largely dictate whether or not treatment is required. If there is an underlying medical condition, then the patient may also have symptoms of this condition.

How is it diagnosed?
The diagnosis is made purely on the patient's history as there is no reliable, objective method of assessing the intensity of the tinnitus. However, the pitch and the level of noise necessary to obscure the tinnitus can be determined and this is important for any subsequent treatment. If the tinnitus affects only one ear, a scan of the inner ear is usually carried out to make sure there is not an underlying acoustic neuroma.

What are the treatment options?

Most people suffering with tinnitus require little more than reassurance that there is no sinister underlying problem. Once reassured, many people find that the impact the tinnitus has on their lives is significantly reduced, since they no longer focus on the problem. Simple steps, such as playing soft music in the background at night, are often helpful. Noise generators or maskers are available to drown out tinnitus and some people who use this technique find that the tinnitus remains less noticeable even after the masker is removed.In those people who have significant hearing loss with the tinnitus, a hearing aid may be beneficial as it tends to increase awareness of background noise, amking the tinnitus less apparent.

Counselling and relaxation play an important role for people with tinnitus, and a number of self-help groups exist.

What is the outlook?

There is no cure for tinnitus in the majority of cases, but the impact that it has on a person's life can be reduced by appropriate advice and reassurance, together with specific aids or treatments in selected cases.

TONSILLITIS
Inflammation of the tonsils.

The tonsils are situated at the back of the mouth and form part of the ring of glandular tissue that protects the upper gastrointestinal tract and airway from infection. Infection in the tonsils is common, especially in children.

What are the causes?

Allergic patients are more prone to tonsil inflammation. Generally, there is a bacterial infection but in some cases the infection is due to a virus. Streptococcal bacteria may permanently reside deep in the tonsils.

What are the symptoms?

Often fever and general malaise precede the onset of a sore throat. The sore throat is the predominant symptom, associated with painful, difficult swallowing. There may be earache and difficulty in opening the mouth. Young children may complain of abdominal pain and may vomit.

The tonsils themselves are swollen and inflamed and there is often pus visible on the surface. There is usually tender lymph gland swelling in the neck. Occasionally, an abscess may form in the tissues adjacent to the tonsil (see Quinsy, p.146) and this exacerbates the pain and difficulty in swallowing and opening the mouth.

What are the treatment options?

The mainstay of treatment is pain relief and plenty of fluids. It is not always necessary to give antibiotics, since the disease is usually self-limiting, but in severe cases recovery may be quicker if antibiotics are given. These are available in tablet form, although it may be necessary to give antibiotics and fluids intravenously if the individual is not able to swallow. Generally, symptoms resolve in less than a week. In people who have recurrent infection, removal of the tonsils should be considered. The criteria for tonsillectomy vary, but five episodes a year for more than two years is a reasonable guide.

VERTIGO
Feelings of dizziness and imbalance.

The balance mechanism involves the complex integration of information from several sources, including the semicircular canals in the inner ear, position-sensitive receptors in the arms and legs and a visual input. These factors are analysed by the brain which coordinates balance and movement. A problem at any point can result in vertigo, so it is vital to look at every aspect of the mechanism in order to identify the cause of the problem.

What are the causes?

Disorders of any part of the balance mechanism can result in vertigo. Inner ear damage results from acute viral infection, as in labyrinthitis (p.138) or from Ménière's disease (p.140). Similarly, disease of the vestibular nerve can cause vertigo and may, for instance, result from a tumour, such as an acoustic neuroma (p.134). There may be disease in the brain itself as a result of a stroke or tumour, or in the spinal cord secondary to multiple sclerosis. There may be disease in the limbs such that the position receptors no longer work correctly. And it is not only disorders of the balance mechanism itself that can cause dizziness.

Disorders of heart and thyroid function, together with other diseases such as anaemia, can all cause dizziness. In addition, certain drugs can cause dizziness. Even after thorough investigation by doctors, a specific diagnosis is not made in about 30 per cent of people.

What are the symptoms?

A wide spectrum of symptoms is included within the term vertigo. Classically, disease of the semicircular canals causes rotational vertigo, whereby the person experiences the sensation of the room spinning around them. This is often made worse by head movements or by closing the eyes, and in some cases may be positional. The vertigo may be sudden or gradual in onset and may be constant or intermittent, depending on the cause. The individual may simply feel a sense of imbalance or other non-specific type of disequilibrium. Depending on the cause of the vertigo, the person may also experience other symptoms originating in the ear. These include hearing loss, tinnitus and occasionally pain or discharge from the ear.

How is it diagnosed?

The vast majority of people are diagnosed on the basis of the history and examination and further investigation is often unnecessary. There is no objective way of reaching a diagnosis in many cases of vertigo. Evidence of disturbance within the balance mechanism can sometimes be seen by observing the eyes (p.109). People suffering from vertigo may also have abnormalities in the way they walk. More detailed assessment of the function of the labyrinth can be performed by looking at the severity and duration of vertigo induced in caloric testing (p.109).

Intermittent, short dizzy spells are likely to be due to poor function in the semicircular canals. An audiogram is also an important part of the investigative process, since many causes of vertigo that originate in the ear are associated with deafness. Measurement of the electrical activity in the part of the brainstem involved in hearing can be used to identify an acoustic neuroma (p.134), but more recently this has been replaced by MRI.

What are the treatment options?

This depends on the cause of the vertigo. Most people with vertigo improve with time. The exceptions to this are those people whose problem has a neurological cause, such as an acoustic neuroma or multiple sclerosis. Many people benefit from specific rehabilitative exercises aimed at encouraging the central nervous system to compensate for the damaged part of the balance mechanism.

Numerous medications are available for the treatment of vertigo, but they are often ineffective and may delay the body's natural compensation. There are treatments for the different conditions causing vertigo. For example, in Ménière's disease an antibiotic to destroy the function of the inner ear is injected into the middle ear. Surgical solutions range from insertion of a grommet to division of the vestibular nerve supplying the balance organs.

LIVING WITH VERTIGO

I was in my late 40s when my Ménière's disease started. I began to have spells when I felt the room spinning. They would come on really quickly, but I could usually tell when I was going to have an attack because I'd get a ringing in my right ear just beforehand.

When it's bad, the attacks can last all day, but fortunately that doesn't happen very often. I know some people who have much worse Ménière's disease than me and they find it really difficult even to go out sometimes. My hearing tends to be a bit variable as well, although it's never been too much of a problem. I do sometimes worry that it might get worse in the long run, but I have noticed that my symptoms have been much better since I cut out coffee and cut down on the amount of salt I put on my food. I miss having anchovies on my pizza, though! I know there are tablets and even an operation that might help, but at the moment my symptoms aren't too bad and I prefer not to take anything. Hopefully it will stay that way.

VOCAL CORD PARALYSIS
A condition in which the vocal cords are unable to move.

The larynx serves a number of purposes, including voice production and protecting the lungs from inhalation of saliva or food (aspiration). These functions are made possible by the ability of the vocal cords to open and close when required. If one or both of the cords become immobile, the individual's lungs are no longer protected from aspiration, the voice will be hoarse and, depending on the position in which the cord is paralysed, the person can, potentially, have difficulty in breathing.

What are the causes?

The movements of the vocal cords are controlled by tiny muscles, which are stimulated to contract by impulses from the brain carried down through the neck to the larynx in the vagus nerve. The left-sided nerve passes right down into the chest before entering the larynx. Disease affecting any part of this pathway can result in a vocal cord paralysis. The most common cause of paralysis is infiltration of the nerve by a tumour, especially in the lung, oesophagus or thyroid gland. In a significant proportion of people, the nerve becomes damaged during surgery on the neck, particularly thyroid surgery. Some cases may be due to damage to the nerve during a road traffic accident or a sporting injury, while others may be the result of a neurological disorder such as a stroke. Around 15 per cent of cases have no attributable cause.

What are the symptoms?
This depends on the position of the vocal cord once paralysed and whether or not both cords are affected. The most common symptoms of a single vocal cord paralysis are hoarseness and an inability to cough adequately. If there is aspiration of food, coughing may follow each mouthful. As a result of foreign material entering the lungs there is a risk of pneumonia. If both vocal cords are paralysed the patient may have difficulty breathing and stridor (p.151). Paralysis on one side may cause the other cord to move gradually towards the midline.

How is it diagnosed?
The patient's history gives the first indication of whether or not there is paralysis. The diagnosis is confirmed by examining the larynx using a flexible endoscope. This is carried out while the individual is awake as the vocal cord movements need to be assessed while the person talks. If there is a paralysis, one or both of the cords will not move.

What are the treatment options?
If only one cord is affected and it is fixed in the midline, most people will not require any treatment, since compensation by the other cord takes place over a period of a few months. If one cord is affected and it is fixed in the open position, compensation may take place, but in some instances there may be persistent problems. In this event, the paralysed cord can be injected with material, usually collagen, in order to push it towards the midline. Alternatively, the fold can be adjusted so that it is positioned closer to the midline.

If there is paralysis of both cords and they are towards the midline, part of one cord can be removed under anaesthetic, most often by using a laser. This opens the airway without totally compromising the voice. There are also several operations that pull the cords away from the midline to make the airway wider. These procedures are successful in around two-thirds of cases. When both cords are paralysed in the open position, the larynx becomes incompetent, the person aspirates food and has a very breathy voice. This is rare and treated by tracheostomy (p.129) to protect the lungs and a laryngectomy (p.130).

WAX BLOCKAGE
A build-up of wax in the ear canal.

Cerumen, or ear wax, is produced when the output of modified sweat glands in the outer part of the ear canal combines with debris formed by dead skin cells. This wax gradually works its way out towards the pinna as a result of the outward growth of the skin lining the ear canal.

What are the causes?
The amount of wax produced varies considerably from person to person. In some instances it can cause blockage of the ear canal, particularly in people who have undergone certain types of ear operation, for example a mastoidectomy, in which the normal anatomical arrangements have been disrupted. However, in the majority of cases the problem of wax blockage is a result of cleaning the ears with cotton buds, which can push the wax deep into the ear canal and can traumatise the skin of the ear canal, hampering its outward growth.

What are the symptoms?
People with wax blockage may experience several symptoms, including a sensation of blockage or earache and mild hearing loss. There may also be a dry cough due to irritation of the vagus nerve which supplies both the skin of the ear canal and the larynx.

What are the treatment options?
Various agents can soften or dissolve ear wax, ranging from olive oil to sodium bicarbonate drops, as well as more specific preparations. They should be instilled into the ear canal with the person lying with the affected ear upwards so that the liquid does not run out. If they are not effective, in most situations the ear can be syringed with warm water by a doctor. If there is an infection or a perforated eardrum, syringing should not be performed. The alternative is wax clearance by an ENT surgeon who will take care not to cause any problems during removal.

Index

Acknowledgments

Carroll & Brown Limited would also like to thank:

Picture researcher
Julia Hanson

Production manager
Karol Davies

Production controller
Nigel Reed

Computer management
Paul Stradling

Indexer
Jill Dormon

3-D anatomy
Mirashade/Matt Gould

Illustrators
Andy Baker, Jacey, Kevin Jones Associates, Debbie Maizels, Mikki Rain, Halli Verrinder, John Woodcock

Photographers
Jules Selmes, David Murray

Photographic sources
GI = Getty Images; IOL = Institute of Laryngology and Otology, University College London; RNTNE = Royal National Throat Nose & Ear Hospital, Royal Free Hampstead NHS Trust; SPL = Science Photo Library; WTMPL= Wellcome Trust Medical Photographic Library

1 Alfred Pasieka/SPL
6 *(left)* Secchi-Lecaque/ Roussel-UCLAF/CNRI/SPL
7 Dr Karl Louna/SPL
8 *(top left)* Mehau Kulyk/SPL
9 GI/Spencer Rowell
10 *(top)* James Stevenson/SPL
11 *(left)* GI/Andy Cox
   (right) Photodisc/Doug Menuez
   (bottom right) CNRI/SPL
12 *(right)* GI/Victoria Blackie
13 Mehau Kulyk/SPL
14 *(left)* Alfred Pasieka/SPL
   (right) David Murray
18 *(bottom left)* Alfred Pasieka/SPL
19 *(top)* Hanan Isachar/Corbis
   (right) David Roberts/SPL
20 *(right)* CNRI/SPL
21 *(bottom)* SPL
22 *(b. left)* Paschal Goetgheluck/SPL
27 *(top left)* Tony Wright/UCL
28 *(bottom)* David Murray
29 *(bottom)* Lauren Shear/SPL

30 *(top)* Clem Haagner, Gallo Images/Corbis
33 *(centre right)* Secchi-Lecaque/ Roussel-UCLAF/CNRI/SPL
35 *(background)* Big Pictures
36 *(b. right)* GI/W & D McIntyre
36-7 GI/Mel Yates
37 *(top)* GI/John Bragg
   (centre) GI/Spencer Rowell
   (bottom) GI/Donovan Reese
38 *(left)* GI/Joe McBride
   (centre) GI/David Chambers
   (right) GI/Michael Dunning
39 GI/Russell Kaye
40 *(left)* Gail Mooney/Corbis
41 *(top right)* Carl & Ann Purcell/Corbis
   (centre right) Richard Hamilton Smith/Corbis
43 Alfred Pasieka/SPL
44-5 *(top)* GI/Joe McBride
48 *(centre)* GI/Laurence Monneret
49 *(left)* Gail Mooney/Corbis
50 Douglas Kirkland/Corbis
55 R.W. Jones/Corbis
56 GI/David Chambers
57 David Murray
58 *(bottom)* Corbis Stock Market
61 *(top)* Robert Llewellyn/Corbis
   (b. left) Patrick Bennett/Corbis
   (b. centre) Photodisc/Steve Mason
   (b. right) GI/Michael Dunning
68 Tony Arruza/Corbis
72 John Birdsall Photography
73 *(top)* GI/Rick Rusing
   (bottom) Corbis/Kevin Fleming
75 Corbis Stockmarket
77 John Noble/Corbis
78 Popperfoto/David Joiner
80 *(centre)* Corbis Stockmarket
   (b. right) Corbis Stockmarket
81 *(b. left)* Neal Preston/Corbis
   (b. right) GI/Charly Franklin
84 Richard Hamilton Smith/Corbis
85 GI/Chris Rawlings
86 GI/Russell Kaye
90 Courtesy HoMedics UK Ltd
91 *(top)* Charles Mauzy/Corbis
   (all others) Eyewire
93 Garden Picture Library/Ron Sutherland/Garden designer Lucy Huntingdon
94 *(left)* Alfred Pasieka/SPL
   (right) Courtesy Dr G Kocjan, University College Hospital, London
95 Andrew Gardner, IOL
98 Alexander Tsiaras/SPL

100-1 AFP/Francois-Xavier Marit
104 Alfred Pasieka/SPL
105 WTMPL
106 Courtesy Karl Storz Endoscopy (UK) Ltd
107 WTMPL
108 *(top)* BSIP, Edwige/SPL
109 Charles East, RNTNE
110 BSIP, Edwige/SPL
111 *(left)* WTMPL
   (right) Charles East, RNTNE
112 *(top)* CC Studio/SPL
   (inset) Manfred Kage/SPL
   (centre left) Chris Priest/SPL
   (centre right) Mehau Kulyk/SPL
113 *(top)* Andrew Gardner, IOL
   (bottom) both Courtesy Dr G Kocjan, University College Hospital, London
114 Dr Karl Louna/SPL
115 *(top)* Custom Medical Stock/SPL
   (bottom) John Griem/SPL
120 *(bottom)* CE
121 *(left)* BSIP, Edwige/SPL
   (centre) Prof Tony Wright, IOL/SPL
122 *(top)* John Hadfield/SPL
   (centre) Jane Shemilt/SPL
   (bottom) BAHA/Entific Medical Systems
123 *(both)* James King-Holmes/SPL
124 *(top)* Charles East, RNTNE
125 *(top and centre)* Andrew Gardner, IOL
   (bottom) Charles East, RNTNE
126 *(top)* Charles East, RNTNE
   (centre) BSIP Boucharlat/SPL
127 Dr P. Marazzi/SPL
128 Dept. of Clinical Radiology, Salisbury District Hospital/SPL
129 WTMPL
131 Ouellette & Theroux, Publiphoto Diffusion/SPL
132 Tim Beddow/SPL
Back cover right WTMPL

Contact details
NHS Direct 0845 4647
www.nhsdirect.nhs.uk

Thanks
Carroll and Brown would like to thank Dr Ian H Flindell, part-time teacher and researcher at the Institute of Sound and Vibration Research at the University of Southampton, and independent consultant in subjective acoustics and environmental noise.

619-005-1